MINDFUL MEDITATION FOR BUSY LIVES

MINDFUL MEDITATION FOR BUSY LIVES

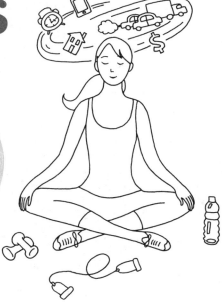

Active Meditation Throughout the Day

Chris Berlow

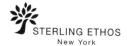

STERLING ETHOS
New York

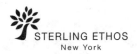

STERLING ETHOS
New York

An Imprint of Sterling Publishing Co., Inc.
1166 Avenue of the Americas
New York, NY 10036

text © 2017 by Chris Berlow
illustrations © 2017 by Alexis Seabrook

ISBN 978-1-4549-2049-6

Distributed in Canada by Sterling Publishing Co., Inc.
c/o Canadian Manda Group, 664 Annette Street
Toronto, Ontario, Canada M6S 2C8
Distributed in the United Kingdom by GMC Distribution Services
Castle Place, 166 High Street, Lewes, East Sussex, England BN7 1XU
Distributed in Australia by NewSouth Books
45 Beach Street, Coogee, NSW 2034, Australia

For information about custom editions, special sales, and premium
and corporate purchases, please contact Sterling Special Sales at 800-
805-5489 or specialsales@sterlingpublishing.com.

Manufactured in Canada

2 4 6 8 10 9 7 5 3 1

www.sterlingpublishing.com

Design by Lorie Pagnozzi

CONTENTS

Section Two: What Do You Love?

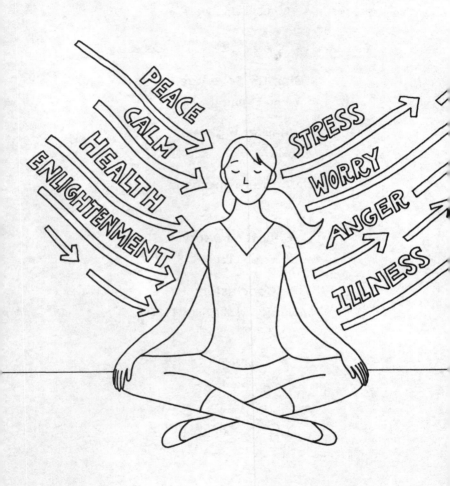

Section One

WHAT IS
MEDITATION?

Chapter 1

Why We All Need to Practice Meditation

It's hard to argue against the idea that our world has become crazy. We are living in such a fast-paced society that it sometimes feels extremely difficult to keep up. With the constant bombardment of social media posts about what seems to be a million changing perspectives, it's no surprise that life seems a bit more complicated than it ever was before. In the general media and news, the majority of content seems negative, focusing on all that is wrong in the world. That's all aside from the daily struggle of balancing work, home, children, hobbies, and everything else. We all experience stress in our lives, and sometimes it seems like there is no outlet to release the frustration and pressure. If stress builds up and we have no way to release it, it will eat away at us. Every day, new scientific studies are published linking a buildup of unspoken stress to physical ailments of every kind—even death.

If all of this sounds pretty negative, that's because it is. Increased stress coupled with a lack of outlets to release this stress is a grave concern of mine, and the challenge is real. Having coached and instructed clients through the personal development company I run with my partners—Empowered Mastery—and through the martial arts I teach and practice, I have seen many people driven to the brink of major illness by a buildup of stress.

When you are stressed, angry, fearful, or downright negative, toxins are released into your system. When those negative emotions have nowhere to go, these toxins build up, your immune system becomes compromised, and your body becomes more vulnerable to physical illness. The truth is that any disease loves stress, anger, and negativity.

Meditation is the solution.

Maybe you've read articles touting the benefits of meditation before. You took a look, sighed, and flipped to the next page—not for you. You're busy. You have commitments. You just don't have the time or focus to sit down and *ommm* your way to inner peace. You have dishes to wash. You have kids to pick up from soccer practice. Your dog just flipped the garbage can over again.

I've got news for you: meditation is still the solution. It's just a matter of looking at meditation as we know it in a different way. You may associate meditation with sitting down and staying silent, but there are other ancient traditions that enable the same kind of mental clarity.

That is exactly what this book is all about: meditation in motion, or what I like to refer to as "active meditation." I define meditation as any activity that totally engages your mind, body, and spirit. When these three elements combine, they create an opportunity for you to "lose yourself" in the moment. In turn, you will receive the many benefits that people all over the world experience through meditation.

People practice meditation for many different reasons. Some do so for religious reasons, some for the calming effect that comes with breathing, and some to enhance their spiritual awareness.

I practice meditation for a multitude of reasons. For one, I benefit from its calming properties. Meditation, whether active or stationary, allows us to slow our brain waves and calm our minds, taking us away from the busyness of life. I also enjoy the sensation of losing myself in my actions. But the greatest gift I gain from meditation is an increased intuition or higher level of awareness.

When I practice meditation, I'm able to see things beyond surface level and find deeper meaning in the actions I perform and the world around me. Those who meditate move beyond the five senses and acquire the opportunity to truly experience inner feelings and emotions; they gain the ability to intuitively study and process situations rather than just react; they are able to prepare for events before they happen and experience a level of calm and confidence like never before; they allow thought energy—

energy stemming from the subconscious mind—to flow freely and effortlessly, and they become more connected to their true selves. This state of heightened intuition can only be achieved through practicing some form of meditation.

....

I must say that I am extremely fortunate in my own physical and spiritual training. For as much as I have gained through the daily practice of active meditation, I know it would not be such an influential part of my life without my own physical and spiritual training in the Korean martial art of tae kwon do. I started my training in 1983 and still actively train and teach every day. I started my instructing career in 1987 under my original tae kwon do instructor, Grandmaster Robert Connolly, and opened my own tae kwon do school with my wife, Kathy, in 1998—the United Martial Arts Centers (UMAC). I made a career teaching tae kwon do and enjoy sharing all that I've learned from my masters and mentors with the students and families that attend my school.

I have had the opportunity to train under my spiritual mentor and tae kwon do instructor, Grandmaster Byung Min Kim, for almost twenty years. He taught me everything I know about meditation. For me, the experience has been life changing, and I am excited to share his teachings with you.

Every Friday, I, with three other master instructors with whom I've been training in the martial arts for many years, see Grandmaster Kim for *dado*. Dado is a traditional Korean tea ceremony where we share quality time, drink special wild green tea, and have discussions based on our personal spiritual training.

During this time, Grandmaster Kim often talks about the term "enlightenment." At one dado session, my training partner, Master Paul Melella, asked what Grandmaster Kim meant by enlightenment. My first inclination was to believe that enlightenment is something mystical and not achievable in my lifetime—something that is only attainable if one were to renounce modern life, live in the mountains, and spend the majority of their days in meditation, silence, and solitude. I was happy to find out that I was wrong.

Grandmaster Kim replied that enlightenment refers to the ability to stay centered, no matter the circumstances. If you are enlightened, nothing can divert you from your center. When we talk about the term "center" in this context, we refer to a place where you are at peace and comfortable in your own skin. A place where you are emotionally stable and things do not easily upset you.

He went on to explain that stress comes from extremes. When someone has the potential to become overly excited, they have an equal potential to become overly angry. In fact, this theory applies to any emotional extremes. Overly happy and excited could become overly sad and depressed. If you've raised a teenage girl, you know exactly what I'm talking about.

For example, I remember one time when my daughter was thirteen. I was giving her a tae kwon do lesson as she prepared for her black belt. I made one comment and gave her a suggestion on a technique, and she started crying. I asked, "Why are you crying?" Her response was priceless: "Dad, I don't know why I'm crying. I just cry for no reason, and I don't like it." I really felt for her that day. Needless to say, she was pretty far off from her center.

Those who achieve enlightenment live stress-free and calm lives; they can ultimately find true happiness. The majority of us will not find and experience true enlightenment in our lifetime; but in truth, it's not really a destination—it's a lifestyle. It may be daunting in a sense to talk about enlightenment as something that is achievable. The objective is to remain as centered as possible when things aren't going your way. By doing so, you will experience less stress and live a more peaceful, harmonious life. In short, the more you experience emotional extremes, the less at peace you will be. The closer you remain to your center, the closer you are to enlightenment.

But how do we achieve enlightenment? Not many people have the ability or desire to change their current lifestyle by foregoing all worldly possessions and living a life of solitude. This approach is potentially the best way to avoid the challenges of life, but it's just not realistic or advisable for the vast majority of people. Therefore, we have to find alternative ways to achieve peace and happiness. Maybe you won't sell your possessions and move to the middle of the forest, but anyone can make an effort to stay as close to their center as possible while life unfolds. There are actions we can all take to avoid the extremes that trigger debilitating stress.

This is where meditation comes into play.

Meditation is the path to enlightenment. It is the most effective tool to train the mind to stay centered, no matter the circumstances. Meditation offers the ability to see things as they are and to look past the surface. Practicing meditation slows brainwaves and allows access to the subconscious mind. According to a 2005 National Science Foundation study, we have up to 60,000 thoughts in any given day in our conscious minds. Meditation filters out the unnecessary, external thoughts and gets to the heart of issues. But what most people don't know is that a variety of activities can be considered meditation.

A perfect example is taking a shower. Have you ever had a moment while taking a shower when ideas just started coming to you? Maybe the solution to a challenge that you were currently facing, or an idea that just came to you out of the blue? Well, showering can be an extremely meditative experience. Imagine:

you are alone with your own thoughts with the warm water flowing down, triggering a comfort that you once felt inside your mother's womb. The act of taking a shower is an extremely relaxing and stress-relieving experience where the deep, imbedded thoughts from your subconscious have an opportunity to come to the surface of your conscious understanding—the craziness of your conscious mind has temporarily subsided.

This is just one example of a daily activity that breaks through the noise of everyday life and into the kind of calm associated with sitting meditation.

The main goal of this book is to provide alternative, non-traditional methods of practicing meditation that will place you on the path toward enlightenment. Meditation comes in many different forms; you may have been meditating all along and didn't even realize it.

Chapter 1 Key Points

- Stress is detrimental to your personal, physical, and mental health.

- Meditation has been reducing and eliminating stress for centuries.

- Enlightenment is the ability to stay centered, no matter the circumstance.

- Meditation is essential in the path toward enlightenment.

Chapter 2

What is Active Meditation?

So what is active meditation?

If you ask most people what meditation is, the image that comes into their mind immediately is someone sitting in what looks like an extremely uncomfortable position, chanting or humming for hours at a time. Honestly, when I started my spiritual development over fifteen years ago, that was exactly what I visualized, too. However, though many practice this kind of meditation, there are also many who practice alternative methods of meditation and achieve similar results.

Many years ago, I was having a great fasting day and had more energy than normal. On a fasting day, I do not eat or drink anything except water. The fast lasts from the night prior to the morning of the following day of the fast. For example, if I started a fast on Tuesday night, I would break the fast on Thursday morning.

During this particular fasting day, I remember feeling great. I taught a sparring class at UMAC and actually participated in addition to teaching. Sparring is incredibly high-energy and strenuous one-on-one training.

I shared my experience with Grandmaster Kim at our weekly training sessions and told him how great I felt while training hard on a fasting day, and he mentioned that sparring is one of the best meditations. Little did I know then that his comment would change my whole perception and understanding of meditation. That moment is when I understood that meditation is not just sitting and breathing rhythmically; it is the total immersion of your body, mind, and spirit into a single activity. A light went off in my brain, and that is how I have introduced meditation to my martial-arts students and personal development clients for many years now.

In one of our training sessions, Grandmaster Kim explained that there are four main types of meditation:

Moving Meditation

Hang Sun meditation is practiced while in motion, focusing on breathing in conjunction with movement and unifying the mind, body, and spirit in a single activity. *Mindful Meditation for Busy Lives* focuses on this form of meditation.

Standing Meditation

Standing meditation focuses on breathing while standing. This is a great form of meditation to practice while waiting in line or in similar situations when one can't sit and meditate.

Sitting Meditation

Sitting meditation is the most practiced form of meditation and is extremely popular. There is a variety of different methods from numerous sources. In Chapter 5, I share how I have been practicing sitting meditation for many years.

Lying-Down Meditation

Lying-down meditation is ideal for working on proper deep breathing. It is also great to practice right before going to sleep. It can help improve the quality of sleep.

....

There are many forms of active meditation, some of which you may already be incorporating in your daily life. However, if you consciously focus on making active meditation more of a priority, you will experience two of its benefits: opportunities for quick rejuvenation, and enhanced performance.

Rejuvenation-Based Meditation

A person can lose himself in an activity when he focuses solely on what he is doing. Think about it. Have you ever been so immersed in an activity that the time just whisked away and, before you knew it, you were done? This often happens when you are engaged in something you thoroughly enjoy.

I remember hiking with my family at the Bryce Canyon National Park in Utah. We only had time for a four-mile hike through the canyons, and I wanted to embrace every moment. My family hiked ahead of me, and I practiced a walking meditation. I walked slowly, looking at every tree and rock formation. I wanted to let it all sink in and embrace every moment. I definitely lost myself in the environment and didn't think of anything else at the moment.

My walk at Bryce Canyon National Park was moving meditation at its best. I wasn't sitting on a pillow for a long period of time—I was actively meditating while walking through the canyons. My mind, body, and spirit were fully embraced in the moment, and nothing else mattered. It was as if I was on a mini rejuvenating vacation from reality, which is one of the benefits of practicing meditation.

Have you ever lost yourself in what you were doing? Sometimes people experience this while working: they become completely engulfed in the moment, even while doing something as mundane as answering e-mails, doing laundry, or simply driving. Some experience this during a sport or activity. For some, it may even happen while walking or playing with their dog.

Any form of meditation other than being still with eyes closed and deep breathing is active meditation. There is no one way of performing active meditation—the only essential part is that you are mentally captivated by what you are doing. And you will feel a sense of rejuvenation as you head back into your day as a result.

Performance-Based Meditation

A person can feel so completely connected to her environment and actions that she feels as if everything is happening flawlessly.

One of the greatest meditative experiences I have witnessed in professional sports happened on May 7, 1995, at the NBA Eastern Conference Semifinals. Reggie Miller of the Indiana Pacers single-handedly defeated the New York Knicks as he scored eight points in eleven seconds. Those eight points ultimately knocked the Knicks out of the playoffs. The next day, newspaper headlines read, triumphantly, "REGGIE MILLER IN THE ZONE!" Here's the kicker: When Reggie Miller was interviewed and asked how he'd done it, he responded by stretching out his huge arms to form a circle and said something along the lines of "The basket was this big." Because of the extent of his concentration, achieving his goals seemed effortless—instead of seeming far away and difficult to attain, the basket was as big as he needed it to be.

What we work for in active meditation is to achieve a state of body, mind, and spirit working as one. Athletes, professionals, children, adults—everyone has the ability to experience the same type of connection as Reggie Miller did that day.

I was once at the 1989 National US Team Trials and in a match with another competitor. I remember vividly that when my opponent attacked, I responded subconsciously. I didn't even realize what had happened until after I had hit my opponent with a back kick. I remember taking a hop back after scoring and thinking, "What in the world just happened?" My mind, body, and spirit worked synergistically, and the result was action without thought. It was almost as if I was looking at the situation from a third-person perspective. It was an awesome experience.

After practicing something for a long time, you eventually master your art. That "art" could be anything in which you have expertise. Through consistent practice and repetition, a skillset develops in your subconscious mind and eventually becomes a permanent, lifelong fixture. Malcolm Gladwell popularized the idea that mastering something requires 10,000 hours of practice, but in many cases, this kind of unconscious mastery is a lifelong commitment.

After practicing a skillset for many years and mastering an art, there are moments where you might feel "on fire" or "in the zone." In the Eastern philosophy of Daoism, this is called "being one with the Dao." These phrases describe the moment when your subconscious takes over and enables you to perform effortlessly. This is a great benefit of, and one of the highest levels of, active meditation. In fact, many people will consider those moments a "spiritual experience"—a moment in time when mind, body, and spirit work together to create perfection, when energy is moving through the body, and it feels like someone else is in control. It is one of the most rewarding sensations that anyone could have.

Benefits of Active Meditation

There are many benefits to be experienced from meditation, no matter the form. Physical health benefits stem from the deep breathing that is required to meditate effectively. The freedom the mind experiences thanks to meditation—both freedom from the thousands of thoughts that filter through the brain every day and freedom to access the subconscious—brings myriad mental health benefits. And there are spiritual benefits from working toward enlightenment, which mostly center around freeing oneself from the pressure and influences of society but vary for each person. Additionally, the benefits of active meditation can provide an unconscious mastery over the environment, which can simulate an out-of-body, third-person perspective. It is a great place to be.

Most people engage in activities for enjoyment or to try something new; they then develop some skills and find themselves forgetting about life for a while. This is what we are working toward with active meditation. For example, think of a really good movie. Have you ever gone to a movie and become so engaged that you completely lost yourself in the film? Sometimes you become so involved that time seems to stop and you forget about everything else. When you leave a captivating movie, you go back to your regular life feeling a bit more refreshed because of the break from reality. That is precisely what meditation—and, by extension, active meditation—is.

Whether you are looking for rejuvenation or improved performance, you will find both in an active meditation practice. Although it does require commitment, diligence, and patience, you will find that regular meditation pays off. In the beginning, certain activities may not feel meditative, because you will be consciously aware of your actions. However, as time goes on, you will become more proficient, allow nature to take its course, and truly experience the benefits of active meditation.

Chapter 2 Key Points:

- There are four main types of meditation: moving, sitting, standing, and lying down.

- Active meditation is your mind, body, and spirit engaged in a single activity.

- The purpose of rejuvenation-based meditation is to "recharge your batteries," in a sense.

- The purpose of performance-based meditation is to excel and achieve better results without conscious thought.

Chapter 3

Proper Breathing

Many of the meditative activities that we will discuss can be greatly enhanced by proper breathing techniques. We all know that breathing is a key element in life. Humans can go weeks without food and days without water, but trying to survive without breathing is a completely different story. When it comes to meditative practices, proper deep breathing is essential, whether it be done while sitting, standing, or lying down, or during moving meditation.

Most people do not breathe properly. Whenever I conduct a seminar on meditation and proper breathing, I always ask the clients and students to take a deep breath. As they do, I see nearly every chest fully expand on the inhale and then retract in on the exhale. This is incorrect for two reasons: first, by expanding the chest, air enters only into the lungs, when really the intake of oxygen should extend to the lower diaphragm; and second, while the lungs are an integral part of the breathing process, it is the lower abdomen that drives the breath.

Have you ever watched a baby sleep? If so, you may have noticed that their breath comes from the lower abdomen. The same is true if you watch a dog or any other animal breathe—you will see their chest remain still and their lower belly move. Over the years, we have come to believe that we have mastered breathing, only to find that we have actually conditioned ourselves to breathe improperly. Even my own personal physician once asked me to take a deep breath at a physical and said I needed to breathe through my chest. To receive the full benefit of oxygen intake, you will need to practice deep breathing. In fact, my mother's pulmonologist taught her the same breathing I practice in my meditation to help her cope with emphysema and Chronic Obstructive Pulmonary Disorder (COPD).

Deep breathing takes place in your lower abdomen—not in your chest. When you inhale, drive your breath by pushing your lower abdomen as far out and as far down as you can. After you have pushed your stomach out all the way—still breathing in all the while—the air will go on to fill your lungs. When you exhale, your stomach should retract in, slow and steady. Practice this for a few minutes. Breathe in slowly and steadily for a count of four, hold the breath for two seconds, and then exhale for a steady count of four. Notice that your chest has nothing to do with the deep-breathing process.

When you initially try this type of breathing, the actions may seem unnatural or cumbersome. It took me a very long time to breathe properly. I found myself questioning whether or not I was deep-breathing correctly for many years after Grandmaster Kim introduced the technique to me back in 1999. It actually felt as if I were performing backward breathing when I first began practicing.

Grandmaster Kim shared a technique with me that helped me understand how to breathe properly, and which I would like to share with you. Close your eyes, and visualize a rope running through your lower abdomen. When you inhale, imagine that the rope is pulling your lower stomach forward. When you exhale, imagine that there is a reverse force pulling the rope from behind you. Visualizing this image through meditation is what helped me learn to breathe properly.

The Benefits of Deep Breathing

Deep breathing has many mental and physical health benefits. Physically, deep breathing brings greater amounts of oxygen into your system, which allows oxygen to flow to the cells throughout your body more efficiently. This in turn increases energy levels, builds muscular strength, increases your metabolism, massages your internal organs, and releases unwanted toxins from your system. In fact, the main reason many people experience headaches is from either lack of water or lack of oxygen. The simple act of taking several deep breaths can clear a headache in minutes. Mentally, breathing aids in calming the mind and in handling stressful situations, plus it gives you mental clarity and provides calming support when emotions are erratic. I am sure everyone has heard someone say "Take a deep breath and calm down."

In the previous chapter, we discussed two types of active meditation: rejuvenating, and performance-based (see pages 14-18). You will find that incorporating proper breathing is essential to achieve the benefits of meditation through activity. The objective is to time your inhale and exhale with whatever it is that you are doing. When you are able to align the two, your mind and body will work harmoniously as one. That is the point when you become more efficient and exertion becomes effortless, driving you toward a spiritual experience where mind, body, and spirit work as one.

I suggest that you practice deep breathing as often as you can. Practice when driving your car, waiting for a meeting, watching television, sitting, standing, lying down—it doesn't matter where, as long as you practice. When you become comfortable with deep breathing and are meditatively engaged in an activity, then proper deep breathing will come to you at a subconscious level without any thought involved.

....

Chapter 3 Key Points:

- Deep breathing benefits your body in the following ways: increases oxygen in the bloodstream; encourages efficient travel of blood cells through the body; raises energy levels; builds muscular strength; heightens metabolism; massages internal organs; and releases unwanted toxins from the body.

- Deep breathing takes place throughout the abdomen, including the belly—not just in the upper chest.

- Practicing upon waking up in the morning or before going to sleep is ideal.

- Use the following steps to practice deep breathing:

  1. Start by practicing this exercise once a day with just five deep inhales and exhales. Increase the number of breaths as time goes on and you become more comfortable.

2. Position yourself by lying flat on your back, arms and legs extended in neutral, comfortable positions.

3. Close your eyes. Visualize a rope pulling your stomach out on the inhale and back in on the exhale.

4. Be consciously aware of your lower abdomen as your practice deep breathing.

5. If lying on your back is uncomfortable for you or you would like a change in position, sit upright with legs crossed and your spine completely erect. Practice deep breathing while maintaining this position.

Chapter 4

We Need to *Calm* Down, Not *Slow* Down

Most people live their lives in one of two modes: reactive, and proactive. When we are reactive, we act after something has acted upon us. When we are proactive, we act first, in anticipation of a corresponding action. However, meditation focuses on a completely different mode: the "being" mode. "Being" is a state where you are able to act without consciously thinking. As awesome as that may sound, it's just about impossible to stay in "being" mode—but a well-developed active meditation practice will help you stay there as much as possible.

As you read about these three modes, please know that everyone is different. The intent here is to see if you, the reader, gravitate toward certain tendencies. The goal is to equip you with tools to understand and experience the benefits of meditation throughout the day.

Reactive Mode

People who live in reactive mode react to circumstances and situations around them. Of course we all have to react at times, because life is unpredictable. However, being constantly defensive and always on guard is not an ideal way to live. People constantly in this mode seem to live by the seat of their pants with little or no routine. People in reactive mode may seem constantly tied up in complex emotional power struggles and always in conflict with one person or another. They may spend a great deal of time on social media reacting to comments and posts. When this kind of intense and frequent reaction is happening, it can be quite challenging to remain calm and centered.

Reactive people tend to feel "scattered" and procrastinate, always waiting until the last minute to accomplish tasks. They're constantly rushing. It is almost as if their lives contain a continuous self-imposed stress that never disappears. I am sure everyone knows this type of person—they very seldom look calm.

I once had a client at Empowered Mastery who was living completely in reactive mode. In fact, he couldn't get out of his own way and was being controlled by everyone and everything around him. He held a demanding upper-level management position, so his compulsion to react to situations as they arose was understandable. When I asked him what he would like to get out of the coaching program in our initial meeting, he said, "To gain control of my life rather than let life control me." He felt that he was constantly one step behind the game and never felt in control professionally or even personally. He had the desire to go to the gym and exercise but couldn't seem to get there. He had the desire to spend more quality time with his family but was never really able to do so.

The first action step I had him take was to put his phone away over the weekend and work on scheduling activities with his family instead of working. These small action steps—pre-planning quality time and living without his phone—were just what he needed. It made him present with his family, which made him feel more fulfilled and happier. The sense of fulfillment in his personal life gave him confidence at work, and he eventually found it easier to schedule some exercise. He became less reactive, more present, and ultimately more productive and happier by learning to control his own schedule.

Are you living in reactive mode? Here are five questions to consider:

1. Do you feel like your schedule controls *you*, instead of your controlling *it*?

2. Are you consistently late for appointments and always apologizing for being late?

3. Are you constantly losing things such as keys, phones, etc.?

4. Do you find yourself not getting back to people when you say you will?

5. Do you feel unproductive in your efforts?

If you answered yes to any of these questions, then it is safe to say that you are living your life in reactive mode. Incorporating a form of meditation into your life will serve you very well.

Proactive Mode

People who live in proactive mode are always thinking ahead. They live their lives in the future, sometimes at the expense of the present. Proactive-mode people have everything pre-planned. They make sure that all the "I's" are dotted and the "T's" are crossed. Details are planned in advance with the hope that everything will go off without a hitch. People as such may be considered "Type A" personalities and are extremely detail-oriented. While this is wonderful for organization and can lend itself to increased productivity and the ability to accomplish goals, there are several negatives to living this way.

Proactive people are extremely productive, high-achieving, and able to accomplish great things. The downside is that they rarely have the ability to turn *off* their engines. Their minds are typically working 24/7, and they rarely get proper rest and rejuvenation. They live ten steps ahead of the game and always plan everything. Stress becomes a frequent issue because, inevitably, obstacles arise and throw a wrench in their well-laid plans. Another challenge for proactive-mode people is that it takes a very long time to decompress. For instance, those living in proactive mode aren't able to really relax on a vacation until the very end, because it's taken them the trip's entire duration to turn off their racing minds—just in time to return to their high-functioning daily lives.

One of the biggest challenges that proactive people face is being present. Because their minds are always on the move and they don't want to miss anything, proactive people find it very hard to break away and free themselves from their immediate problems.

I once had a very dedicated student in our martial-arts fitness kickboxing program. She was very much a proactive, type-A personality. In fact, every time I gave the students a rest, she would rush to her phone, check her e-mails to see what she had missed, and handle an issue if there was one. Her phone held her captive.

After observing this for some time, my initial solution was to eliminate all rests and breaks, so we would train straight through the practice without stopping. It actually worked for a while, until this student and I had a conversation about why I had eliminated the breaks. Of course, my students loved the intense training, but I had made my decision because she needed a break from her phone. She wasn't giving herself the opportunity to be completely engaged in her training and therefore wasn't benefiting thoroughly. Yes, she was getting a good physical workout, but she wasn't rejuvenating her mind because her focus was always half on class and half on work. Training in martial arts and kickboxing is meant to be an escape—if you are on your phone throughout the workout, then you're depriving yourself of one of its greatest benefits. I suggested she give herself the gift of time and turn off her phone so she could have a chance to recharge her batteries.

As a result of our conversation—and many more after—she changed her focus to traditional martial-arts training and achieved a black belt. She is now training to become an instructor and never brings her phone to class. She found balance and freedom from what was holding her back the most. Her proactive personality was actually stifling her productivity because she wasn't giving herself an opportunity to recharge her batteries. If you are always connected to your smartphone during activities, put it aside and learn to give yourself the gift of time just as my student has.

Are you living in proactive mode? Here are four questions to consider:

1. Do you find yourself over-scheduling and fitting as much as you can in each day?

2. Do you over-analyze situations and find it hard to come to a decision?

3. Are you always with your smartphone and have a hard time disconnecting from social media?

4. Do you find yourself striving to be perfect in everything you do? And when you don't achieve perfection, do you feel frustrated?

Being Mode

A while back, I was attending a life-coaching certification program with Bob Proctor, one of the foremost leaders in personal development. He said something very powerful at the seminar that made complete sense regarding many of today's challenges. He explained that life is getting faster and faster, and most people have a hard time keeping up. A lot of people are stressed, always rushing to keep pace (even though that's virtually impossible) and have begun to expect instant gratification. He said, "It's not that people need to slow down—because there is no slowing down. They need to *calm* down." That completely resonated with me and reinforced my belief in the need for meditation and the practice of mindful activities.

Many people work hard just to get by, reacting to situations as they arise, while others plan every aspect of their lives and barely live in the present. Neither type of person is really able to calm down, because they live outside of their current reality. "Being mode" is when people are able to stay present, balance the different aspects of life, and appreciate what is happening in the moment. Then—and only then—will they have the ability to calm down, and just "be." When you are able to just "be," you can watch life unfold in front of you and observe it as if from a third-person perspective; you are no longer in the craziness of life but rather are above it.

To achieve this heightened level of awareness, you need to be more present and mindful of the daily activities of life. Find the ability to turn off your phone and only check it at times that will not affect the moment. Train yourself not to worry about what you might be missing; know that you can handle whatever may come your way. The confidence this will bring is true freedom. You will be in control of your life instead of life being in control of *you*. That is personal power.

Twenty years ago, cell phones were clunky and expensive, and the Internet was just gaining traction. Remember going out to dinner without a phone? Twenty years ago, you had to use a pay-phone to check in with your children. Back then, people lived in body, mind, and spirit without the distractions of so many "things." That was an era when society was not held captive by technology. Those were simpler times, when personal connection was the norm.

Leave your phone in the car while running errands—you'll be surprised and gratified by the results.

Thinking: Without your phone, you'll find yourself contemplating what's important to you. You'll find that it's considerably easier to direct your attention to what is necessary without distraction. As a result, your mind will begin forming solutions for challenges you may be facing, like answers for personal and business issues.

Communicating: Being away from your phone will give you an opportunity to engage with people, make eye contact, and be genuinely thankful for their service. You'll find that this goes a very long way to making you feel more connected to your community. When you have an opportunity to disconnect from the phone for a little while, you will be amazed at how productive you may be.

Some of you may have come to the realization that you are living either reactively or proactively. Don't worry: here are some strategies to implement that will help you live in "being" mode and experience holistically what life has to offer.

If You're Reactive

If you are in reactive mode, here are some action steps to take to help reclaim balance, calm down, and become more present.

- Give yourself fifteen minutes of extra lead time to get where you are going.

- Plan your day in the morning, and do your best to time-block the important appointments and responsibilities you have.

- Only check your smart phone and social media outside of the time blocks, when you are free.

- Be willing to leave your phone off and have phone-free days. Don't worry—the world will not fall down around you.

....

If You're Proactive

If you live in proactive mode and have a hard time not thinking of the future and planning every part of your life, here are some action steps to help you de-stress and live more presently.

- Since you are efficient with your time, be sure to block out some time to do something that you thoroughly enjoy.

- When you find that activity, don't pick up the phone until you finish.

- When you are with your family or people you care about, engage in genuine conversation—and, again, leave your device out of it.

....

At the end of your days, you are going to leave this world with what you were born with: nothing. You can't take material items or money with you to the grave; you will be traveling solo at the end. The one and only thing you could leave behind is a legacy. That legacy is the relationships you have formed and the time you have spent with the people you care for most.

I urge you to be as present and mindful as possible. Do not miss out on the present and lose memories that will last a life-time. Quality of life is not measured by what you have, but by who you are and what you mean to others. The phrase "live life to the fullest" means to enjoy all that life has to offer in the present. That is the essence of the next chapter: mindfulness.

Chapter 4 Key Points

- Reactive mode is a state of mind in which you feel you are a few steps behind in all that you do.

- Proactive mode is a state of mind in which you plan everything in advance, prepare for the future, and find it hard to calm down.

- "Being" mode is a state of mind in which you are present in the moment and aware of what is going on at all times.

Chapter 5

Mindfulness

When I was just conceptualizing this book, I had a conversation with one of my martial-arts mentors, Sensei Joe Joe, during a training session. I had been practicing sitting meditation and alternative methods of meditation for many years by that point, and I was curious to hear how Sensei Joe Joe had integrated meditation into his practice.

Sensei Joe Joe is a lifelong martial artist; he was born and raised in Japan and brought up around Japanese martial arts, including karate, kobudo, and judo. He knew at a very young age that he wanted to teach karate as a profession. He lives a very simple life of training and teaching martial arts. He doesn't even have a cell phone and is very secluded from modern-day technology.

Sensei Joe Joe mentioned that it is very hard to sit and practice meditation for some people. He told me, "In my culture, it is all about Zen. Zen is being present and mindful in what you are doing at the moment—to have a present mind." He added that when he and his wife drink coffee, they are embracing the moment of time in which they are drinking coffee and appreciate every aspect of the experience. When he is outside, he is not just walking to his destination, but is appreciating the walk and all that is around him. Sensei Joe Joe believes that it is important to take the time to recognize the beauty that is around him in every moment. He mentioned that this is why he chooses not to have a cell phone: he doesn't want to be distracted from the moment.

The most interesting thing about our conversation was not the conversation itself, but the timing of it. The conversation organically occurred within one week of my decision to write this book. Life is full of amazing coincidences—or maybe there are no coincidences at all and everything is meant to be. It was a perfect example of "being" mode. If we were not completely engaged in our conversation and aware of our words, meanings, and environment, we wouldn't have had that conversation in the first place. You will be amazed by what comes your way when you are more aware of the present.

I remember when Grandmaster Kim first introduced me, and the other masters I train with, to Korean wild green tea. We were at a dado ceremony, and I found it very powerful and meaning-ful. I wanted to share the experience with my top adult students, so I purchased the tea and a set, and I held my first dado session.

One of the most special parts of the tea ceremony is the gift of shared time: being present with the company around you as you experience a wonderful tea that nature has provided. As we were having tea and waiting for the water to cool to a specific temperature, one of my students said, "Sir, if you put the water over here, it will cool faster." I explained to him that the whole idea is not to speed through the tea-brewing process, but to appreciate the time together and savor the taste of the tea.

During Grandmaster Kim's training sessions, there are no cell phones, no computers, no distractions; just shared time. We are all fully present and mindful of the conversation and the company.

Another timely striking moment that also emphasizes the power of mindfulness occurred during a dado session with Grandmaster Kim a few months after I began writing this book. During the session, he explained that drinking tea offers many more benefits than just the physical benefits of drinking it. For example, when he was pouring the tea, he waited until the very last drop spilled out of the spout, explaining that this is a lesson in patience. The residue in the bottom of the cup, which is thrown away, represents bad habits. Grandmaster Kim also explained the importance of savoring each and every sip and appreciating the experience and taste as you drink the tea. The point is that, during this ritual, one is 100 percent present and mindful of every action and moment.

Mindfulness is not a new phenomenon but has been practiced

since the beginning of recorded time. While it may have been easier back then because there were no distractions like cell phones, there are still numerous mentions of the importance of being fully present in a variety of cultures. Nearly every philosophy and religion has integrated the practice and belief in the power of mindfulness. In a January 13, 2015 article featured in the *Huffington Post*, author Sarah Rudel Beach writes:

> Virtually every spiritual tradition has practices for mindful contemplation and silence, and direct awareness of experience, such as Catholic centering prayer, Buddhist meditation, the Jewish Shabbat or Sufi mysticism. Many secular philosophies incorporate these teachings as well. The Roman Stoic philosophers Seneca, Epictetus and Marcus Aurelius advocated an approach to life that today we might label as mindfulness; Aurelius wrote, "Our perturbations come only from the opinion which is within."

For example, mindfulness is the true essence of Buddhism. When the Buddha was asked, "Sir, what do you and your monks practice?" he replied, "We sit, we walk, and we eat." The individual said, "But, sir, everyone sits, walks, and eats." The Buddha responded: "When we sit, we *know* we are sitting, we *know* we are walking. When we eat, we *know* we are eating."

The greatest aspect of mindfulness is that it seems to slow down time. If you are present and completely in tune with reality, then time will slow and make that moment feel infinite. Therefore the mind won't be cluttered with concerns about the future or the past—all that exists is the present. Once your mind wanders to the future or the past, then the eternity of the moment is lost. When you practice mindfulness, a greater appreciation and gratitude will fill your mind, heart, and soul, and you will find true beauty in your actions.

....

Chapter 5 Key Points:

- Mindfulness is being fully present and aware of your actions at every moment.

- Tips to help develop mindfulness:

  1. Savor every flavor in every sip or bite that you take.

  2. When performing a task, be sure to focus only on the task at hand, and move on to the next only after the first is completed.

  3. Take the time to look outside and recognize five beautiful things about nature around you.

4. Close your eyes and listen to the sounds of nature for five minutes.

5. When engaged in conversation, listen to everything that is said. Don't just "hear"—listen.

6. Repeatedly say to yourself, "I appreciate the now" when you find your mind wandering.

Chapter 6

Time

I don't believe there is anything more valuable or important in life than time. The most common objection for someone to do anything new is the classic line, "I would, if I had the time. . . ." The truth is that everyone has the time if they choose to make a new activity a priority. That goes for all forms of meditation, whether active or sitting.

On that note, a favorite meditation saying passed down in the Buddhist tradition is: "Everyone should meditate for twenty minutes. If you don't have time, you should meditate for an hour." This says it all. Everyone needs to find time to take care of themselves. If you don't make your personal development a priority, it will be extremely difficult to make strides in other areas of your life.

Many years ago, while I was having tea with Grandmaster Kim, the topic of time came up. He asked us to write a paper on our beliefs when it comes to managing our time. Here is what I submitted:

Time is the most valuable commodity we have in our lives. It ticks away with every breath we take and every moment we spend. It's not like we can add two more hours to every day to spend more time doing what we want. A twenty-six-hour day would be nice, but it's not going to happen. I've often heard from parents of tae kwon do students and from prospective adult students that they would train if they had more time. My thoughts on this matter are as follows:

Everyone has the ability to choose how and where they spend their time. We all have twenty-four hours in a day and could choose to spend it however we wish. Everyone has the gift and power to do so. If someone is not happy with how they spend their time, then they have to do something about it. They have to prioritize and arrange their day in a way that allows them to do what they want. A great way to explain this is the difference between spending *time and* wasting *time.*

Spending Time: *Spending time is allotting time to do the things that you want to do with the people you want to be with. For example, when I am with all of you—my fellow master instructors—training and having tea, there is nothing in this world that I would rather be doing at that moment, so therefore I am spending my time wisely. When I am with my family, I am spending my time wisely. When I am at the UMAC teaching class, I am spending* *my time wisely.* Spending *time is doing what you choose with the people you want to be with.*

Wasting Time: *Wasting time is the opposite of spending time. If I am forced into an activity I have no desire to do or have to spend time with people I prefer not to see, then that is wasted time. Other examples of wasting time include conversing with people trying to sell something to you that you don't want; attempting an act or skill that is out of your comfort zone and that you know, in your heart, will not help you achieve your goals; or spending time with those who take positive energy out of you and do not provide productive relationships. If the action or relationship is a huge burden and wears you down mentally and emotionally without any good feelings in return, then you are wasting your time. If you're passing time with a close friend or family member who you love very much, then that is time well spent.*

We have the ability to utilize our time and spend it wisely—not waste it. We can do this by embracing everything that happens throughout the day. As you are going through the day, try to make other people happy. Share your love for life, say "thank you" to a cashier, give them the gift of your time by looking at them and saying, "Have a great day." That is spending time wisely, even though it may not be productive. Also, we should practice being completely present at all times and looking at all situations—positive or negative, both successes and hardships—as training to improve our selves. If we look at every situation in our lives as an opportunity to improve, we are spending our time wisely.

Another way to create more time in our lives is to be more focused. If you are in the office designing a flyer and are constantly getting distracted by phone calls, e-mails, and interruptions, that flyer may take you three hours to complete. However, if you were completely focused without disruptions, the flyer may take only forty-five minutes. Maximize your time by focusing solely on what you would like to accomplish so you'll have more time to spend on other things.

I explain to my children and many of my students that homework could take a half hour, or it could take two hours. If you focus, it will take you a half hour, and if you leave yourself vulnerable to distractions, it will take you two hours. Remember that if you organize your time differently, you could spend that extra hour and a half doing what you want.

All in all, you are in charge of your success. You can create as much time as you like for what you want, or you can constantly feel rushed. Work should not feel like an obligation—it should be fun. Many people do not like their careers, and I feel for them. When I had to work in a job I didn't enjoy, I reminded myself how fortunate I was for the ability to provide for my family. Attitude has a tremendous impact on how you feel about your time.

Whatever job you have should be viewed as a fun, exciting career. Having the attitude of gratitude will only give you more opportunities for the future. Either you need to change your perspective on work or find a career that matches your passion. Remember, the goal is to spend time wisely, not watch it wither away. I personally never say I have to go to work on any given day. I say that I am going to play. That is because I get to do what I love every day with people I care about tremendously. What better life is there? We, as master instructors, spend every day living in and sharing our passion with others. We must share our enthusiasm for tae kwon do with others and let them know that they could live their lives to the fullest if they incorporate our concepts and philosophies. If we can do that successfully, then our students will see that martial-arts training is spending time and is essential to getting the most out of life.

A final thought: Prioritize your time. If you have set meaningful goals and they are strong in your mind, you will do whatever it takes to achieve them. If the goal

is to meditate every morning and every night and it is
important enough to you, you will make it happen—you
will rearrange your schedule to do so. If it is not important
to you, you won't make it happen.

—*Master Chris Berlow*

Until everyone who reads this book believes that their meditation practice is time well spent, they will never reap the benefits. After meditation, whether stationary or active, I always feel better and mentally rejuvenated with a sense of inner peace and a clear mind. Everyone can experience the same, as long as they block special time every day to practice some form of meditation.

Chapter 6 Key Points

- Personal development must be a priority; otherwise, it is extremely difficult to make strides in other areas of life.

- *Spending* time is allotting time to do the things that you want to do with the people you want to be with.

- *Wasting* time is being forced into an activity one has no desire to do or with people one prefers not to see.

- *Spend* time more wisely by analyzing your calendar and determining whether scheduled tasks are worth your time; allocating time for distraction-free meditation; and turning your phone and access to social media off.

- Once time is gone, you will never get it back—treat your time as a priceless treasure.

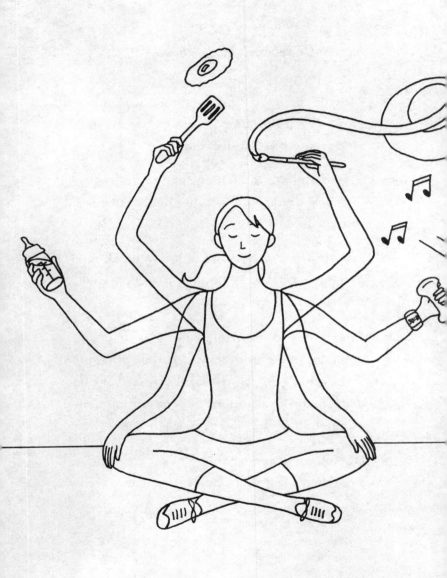

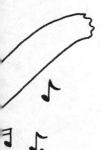

Section Two

WHAT DO YOU LOVE?

Chapter 7

Acquire the Ability to Meditate

I believe that anything can have a meditative component to it. Active meditation is about engaging in an activity that totally engulfs your mind, body, and spirit. But it cannot be forced. The more you force an experience with the expectation that it will become a form of meditation, then the less likely it will happen. Don't confuse meditation with hard work. A key benefit of any meditative experience—aside from the mental escape from reality that meditation provides—is the ability to relax. Relaxation is a key element that cannot be overlooked. When you relax, you allow thought energy to flow to and through you easily and effortlessly without resistance. When you resist, your body and mind tighten up, and the energy stops dead in its tracks. That is why a shower is a wonderful meditative experience. In the shower, you are relaxed, so your thought energy flows to and through you without resistance. Add stress, anxiety, doubt, tension, frustration, and the energy flow will stop immediately.

When you are learning a new skillset or hobby, there is typically a learning curve. On the learning curve will be feelings of frustration, doubt, and some other negative emotions. These emotions are real; they will negatively affect the meditative benefit you seek. In the beginning, you may find it difficult to get past these feelings; but if you practice and gain confidence through repetition, you will begin to see consistent meditative benefits.

My wife Kathy and I love snowboarding. We are avid snowboarders and have a little place in Stowe, Vermont. We love it there, and we often bring our whole family to enjoy the sport that has become a passion for most of us. Snowboarding itself is not inherently relaxing, but it does provide meditative benefits. When I am snowboarding, I am thinking about nothing else in life except the experience. The trails I prefer are typically in the backcountry and involve going down the most technical terrain on the mountain, so the amount of concentration and focus it takes to conquer the backcountry elements and stunts keeps my mind free from all outside distraction. If I am not mindful of the moment and aware of my surroundings, serious injury could occur.

I am able to escape from my current reality through challenging myself mentally, physically, and spiritually to accomplish things I was at one time nervous about: flying through the backcountry, dodging natural obstacles such as trees, rocks, and ledges, and finding the most challenging terrain within my scope of ability.

My snowboarding experience, however, is very different from my wife's. My experience is more of a performance-based meditation (see page 16). On the other hand, Kathy experiences a rejuvenation-based meditation (see page 14) when she snowboards. Kathy is happy going down the same trail over and over again. On her white snowboard with its pink underside, she melts into the mountain, floating down without having to pay close attention to details. She sometimes listens to a favorite playlist. She is totally in her own world and can relax completely. Snowboarding requires the boarder to carve the direction in which he or she is going, edge to edge, in a nice half-moon pattern. The more you lean into your edge, the easier the turn and the less effort required. When Kathy rides down the mountain, she is a perfect example of beauty and art in motion. Her technical mastery over the action of snowboarding, as well as the fact that she has repeated the same trail many times, allows her to perform the action perfectly without thinking.

It wasn't always like that for Kathy. When she first started, she was so frustrated. She fell all the time and could not master her turns. When she first started learning, she had so many bruises on her backside that it looked like an image of the world map. But she was so perseverant that she wanted to get out there even when she was injured and continued to snowboard regardless of her injuries. When Kathy broke her wrist, even the doctor was impressed by her stubbornness—he eventually acknowledged that she was going to get back out there even though he advised her not to, so instead of recommending bed rest, he just gave her an extra-strong cast.

It was through diligent practice and hard work that Kathy acquired the skills to snowboard at an expert level. She always loved snowboarding, but now she has added the benefit of being able to enjoy it at a meditative level. She can perform the basic actions of snowboarding without thinking about it consciously. It didn't come easy, and it took a lot to get there.

With any new activity, interest, or passion, you will have to practice before you can enjoy it as a meditation. After you've mastered whatever skill you choose, you'll find yourself benefiting just from the repetition of it—your thoughts will be completely immersed in the activity. However, it may take some time (and a lot of practice) before you can relax completely.

People find sanctuary in a number of different activities. There is no one activity better than another; it really comes down to interests. In the next few chapters, we will explore different activities, hobbies, and interests, and I will share expert opinions on why and how those specific activities are great forms of meditation. What you'll learn is that it doesn't really matter what activity or hobby you engage in—what matters is that you are able to experience the benefits of meditation provided by each one of them.

....

Chapter 7 Key Points

- No matter what you choose as a hobby or interest, know that there will be a learning curve before you can experience meditative benefits.

- In a challenging activity—such as snowboarding in the backcountry—the intense focus and attention to detail can provide performance-based meditative benefits.

- In a rhythmic, proficient activity—such as snowboarding on easier, more familiar trails—the ability to engage without thought can provide rejuvenation-based meditative benefits.

....

Chapter 8

Mindful Activities:
Running/Swimming/Biking

On the day I wrote this chapter, my older brother John celebrated his fiftieth birthday. For the first forty-five years of his life, he was definitely not what you might call the athletic type. He always had an adventurous spirit and loved the outdoors and hiking, but was never one to partake in endurance activities. Well, something changed around his forty-fifth birthday. He started running, then he started riding a bicycle, and then he even started to swim. He found such great satisfaction and mental release through the endurance activities that he started working toward becoming a triathlete.

As a paramedic for the local fire department, his sporadic schedule sometimes left him with blocks of uninterrupted time, which he devoted to training. His first goal was to be able to call himself a triathlete. Once he completed his first sprint triathlon (short distance), he increased the distances and competed in longer and more rigorous events. He trained to run a half marathon and completed a full marathon within a year of when he started his training. Since then, he has completed a half-Ironman Triathlon and is in training for a full-Ironman Triathlon in the near future.

I've never had the same passion for endurance training, although I do love intense physical activities like martial arts and mountain biking. My brother, however, inspired me to try endurance events, so I did. First, I trained for an off-road sprint triathlon called XTERRA. I discovered I loved running in the woods, and I already loved mountain biking, so all I needed to learn was how to swim competitively. So I did. I competed in the XTERRA, then, inspired by my progress, started running more and more, picked up a road bike, swam more, biked more, ran more—and suddenly, I was an endurance athlete. I completed my first full marathon in April 2015. My initial reasons for doing all this were simple: I wanted to spend more time with my brother. To this day, we still train together when we have a chance.

Running

Being with my brother motivated me to run more than any personal desire could—in fact, running in and of itself isn't usually pleasurable to me. Although there are days where my run feels great and I experience its meditative benefits, running is a bit challenging for me. I've had problems with injuries to my feet because of my tae kwon do practice, so I can really never let my thoughts wander because of the pain. After getting properly fitted with the right pair of running shoes, I've been able to enjoy running more, but I just can't enjoy it for itself alone.

My business partner and co-founder in Empowered Mastery, Rick Wollman, started running in 1985 and is still at it today. The beauty of Rick's passion for running is that he doesn't do it for a goal or for medals, not to compete in a race, and not even to spend time with running partners—he does it for the pure love of running.

Rick started running because his brother Sandy was completing marathons and Ironman Triathlons. Sandy said to Rick, "You have nothing to do, so go out for a run." Rick heeded his older brother's advice, borrowed his roommate's running shoes, and went on his first half-hour run. Little did he know that that would be the start of a thirty-year journey on which he has logged over 25,000 miles.

Christopher McDougall's book *Born to Run: A Hidden Tribe, Superathletes, and the Greatest Race the World Has Never Seen* is a book that Rick highly recommended I read. In *Born to Run*, a group of people runs in a secret ultra-endurance race deep in Mexico's Cotton Canyons. The only female of the group, Jenny Shelton, offered a perfect description of running as a form of meditation as she reflected on the extreme adventure. "When I'm out on a long run, the only thing in life that matters is finishing. For once my brain isn't going 'blah, blah, blah, blah.' Everything quiets down, and the only thing going on is pure flow. It's just me and the movement and the motion. That's what I love—just being a barbarian running through the woods."

Like Jenny, Rick eventually realized that running had become his own personal form of meditation. He was never aware of this until he heard me speak about running as a form of meditation at one of Empowered Mastery's seminars. I interviewed him prior to writing this book, and he told me:

"I feel my thoughts going through me as I am running. Running has become a form of meditation because it is when I am in my most relaxed state. Ideas come to me mostly because I am consciously aware of my thoughts when I am running. Good ideas come into play, and I am frequently reminded of things that I need to do or haven't done yet," he said.

Rick mentioned that he has achieved a "runner's high" many times and considered it to be an out-of-body experience. A runner's high is a state of being in which one experiences running at a spiritual level with no physical exertion whatsoever.

Rick shared an example of runner's high with me. He was in Boston on business and out for a run at 5:00 A.M. Rick looks at running as perfect preparation for a day's meetings and seminars with clients. He claims it helps him perform at a higher level because he uses his time running as an opportunity to mentally leaf through everything he has to do for the day. "If you could think about all that you have to do for the day while you're running, you'll have it down pat," says Rick.

It was dark at five o'clock in the morning. Rick's plan was to run in one direction for forty-five minutes, then turn around and come back to his hotel. During the run, a woman ran past him on the same path. Now, most people's ego and pride kick into gear when being passed by another runner, and Rick is no different. Being a competitive person, Rick stepped up his pace. He successfully passed her, but instead of slowing down and resuming his usual stride, Rick kept up the same pace. He knocked out the last four miles in no time and felt stronger at the end of the run than when he started. He cites that as a perfect example of runner's high. During our interview, Rick provided some great advice for those looking to take up running.

"Don't set goals. If you set goals, you will only be running for the sense of accomplishment, and that will defeat the purpose. Just do it for the pure enjoyment of running. Put on the running shoes and start to run at a very slow pace, but be sure to do it for fun," he suggested.

Rick was adamant about simply running for fun and not for a goal. The reason for this is that so many people develop stress and anxiety because they set goals that may or may not be achievable. While having goals can provide inspiration, the pressure that comes with achieving the goal detracts from the beauty and moment of the experiences. Know that running may not be fun in the beginning, but if you keep at it, you could experience the elusive runner's high.

Rick also added that you should invest in a good pair of running shoes after you've made running a habit. I highly recommend you go to a running store, where a specialist can properly fit you for running shoes. They also take previous injuries like mine into account and can give you advice for training and competing.

Rick sees running as a form of meditation, but this can be true for all endurance sports. When an action is steadily repeated for long periods, your mind can take a backseat to what your body is doing. That is where meditative experiences start.

Action Steps to Begin Running

1. Just do it! Throw on a pair of running shoes and run for ten or fifteen minutes.

2. Start out slow, and don't push yourself too much in the beginning.

3. Invest in a good pair of running shoes by going to a running store to get properly fitted. (This makes a world of difference.)

4. Find peaceful and quiet places to run that are convenient.

5. Develop a music playlist to help you zone out while running.

6. Always stretch after you run, and listen to your body—stop if you experience pain.

7. Run for fun and enjoy.

....

Foster a Meditative Environment While Running:

* Relax. Be consciously aware of relaxing your muscles, especially your shoulders.

* Appreciate your surroundings when running in a quiet or outdoor area, pausing to do so if need be.

* Be aware of your body. Feel and experience the rhythm of each stride that you take.

* Pay attention to your breathing. If you are breathing too heavily, slow down until your breathing coordinates with your strides. For example, inhale with two strides, and then exhale with two strides.

....

Swimming

There is no one who knows more about swimming than Rick's older brother, Sandy Wollman. He completed the 2.4-mile swim, 112-mile bike ride, and 26.2-mile run that comprise the Ironman Triathlon—one of the most physically and mentally demanding feats that anyone could accomplish. After participating in *three* Ironman Triathlons, Sandy decided to accept the invitation for an ultra-endurance swim and swam around the island of Manhattan. After completing the nine-hour swim, he craved a greater challenge, so he made a commitment to swim across the English Channel, from the coast of England to the coast of France. According to the Channel Swimming Association, to cross the English Channel is to face a twenty-one-mile (thirty-two-kilometer) open-water swim across ever-changing tides and currents.

When talking to Sandy about the swim, he told me it was the most challenging accomplishment of his life and one he will remember until his very last breath. He completed the swim in thirteen hours and six minutes, and was the 470th person in history to successfully complete the challenge—one with a meager 10-percent success rate.

Sandy attributes his success to two things: staying positive and respecting the water. For instance, before beginning the English Channel swim, he cracked open a bottle of champagne and dumped it into the water to share with the ancient sea god, Poseidon.

During our discussion, Sandy reflected on how swimming

could be an effective form of meditation. He shared that while he was swimming, he was at first able to zone out because there was very little external stimulation—it was only him and the open sea. His mantras during his swim were "one stroke at a time" and "just one more stroke," which he repeated throughout the ultra-endurance swim. To swim 21 miles across the tumultuous waters of the English Channel while fighting obstacles like sea creatures, hypothermia, fatigue, and rolling tides, one definitely needs to reach a meditative state.

One story that Sandy shared during our conversation stuck out to me. He described a different kind of meditation he experienced while swimming, one I have never heard of before, called "anger meditation." He experienced this in what he called the "worst hour" of the swim. He was behind schedule due to the change in tides, and the captain of the boat following him—in case of an emergency—let him know that he had to swim faster than ever before for the next hour. He was already tired but now had to give maximum effort or else extend his swim another three hours.

The captain's method of encouragement, although unorthodox, was very effective—he told Sandy: "If you miss the tide, you'll add three hours to your swim. For the next hour, swim faster than you have all day" before hitting him on the head with a stick. The captain declared that he would not feed Sandy or give him a break until he finished the swim, and then proceeded to throw chicken bones at him.

While this may sound cruel, it was actually a mind game. The captain was diverting Sandy's attention away from the agony of the swim by giving him a new focus: "hating" the captain. In Sandy's words, ". . . the best thing he could have done was to get me angry."

But how, exactly, did Sandy achieve meditation and mindfulness at all during his challenge?

Mindful swimming requires the effortless coordination of breath and stroke to the point when the swim becomes rhythmic and automatic instead of concentrated effort. The timing of breath with the stroke is key for maximum efficiency. In swimming, it is not the effort that matters, but the glide—where you create less resistance against the water. The better you time the movement of your body with the positioning and repositioning of each stroke, the more glide you will have. Some swimmers alternate which side of their stroke they breathe on, and some prefer to breathe on one side only. Some breathe on every stroke, whereas others may breathe on every third stroke. The preference is personal, but it is highly recommended that you receive training from a professional to ensure proper and safe technique.

Anyone looking into swimming as a form of meditation must respect the water. Don't take anything for granted, and be sure to learn from a professional if you don't feel confident. To maximize the meditative element, be sure to slow down your stroke and align it with your breathing. Remember, efficient swimming is key, and when you relax into a steady rhythm, you will easily be able to zone out during your swim. There's no need to swim the English Channel to experience the meditative benefits of swimming.

....

Action Steps to Begin Swimming

1. Research a local venue where you can swim with lifeguards on duty.

2. Take lessons to ensure proper technique and breathing.

3. Start out slow, and don't push yourself too much in the beginning.

4. Respect the water.

....

Foster a Meditative Environment While Swimming:

• Relax. Consciously be aware of relaxing your muscles, especially your shoulders.

- Breathe deeply and with purpose. Focus on timing your breathing with your strokes.

- Achieve effortlessness. Work on timing your strokes and breathing in order to glide through the water effortlessly.

- Be aware of your body—swimming is a total body experience. Practice paying attention to all the moving parts and streamlining your motions.

Biking

As a child in my pre-martial arts days, I spent every moment I could on my BMX bicycle. I loved to ride. I would get home from school, hop on the bike with a friend, and head to the local aqueducts and trails. We would ride for hours until we had to get back home for dinner. As I grew older, my passion for martial-arts training replaced my passion for riding, though I didn't stop biking—my bicycle became a way to get to my training.

Twenty years later, a good friend of mine pulled into my martial arts school all muddy with a dirty mountain bike on the back of his car. He said he had gone mountain biking. I asked if I could join him one day, and once my tires hit the trails, I was hooked! I was back on the trails and felt as if I were a twelve years old again.

Since my reintroduction to biking fifteen years ago, I have been an avid mountain biker and have competed at the local and national level. I have raced cross-country. I've also done downhill riding, where you need to take a ski lift to get to the trails. Mostly, I enjoy the time spent with good friends flying through the woods on our bikes, playing on obstacles, and acting like twelve-year-old adults.

Mountain biking is both invigorating and calming. It's invigorating in the same way as backcountry snowboarding, which challenges my body and mind and keeps my adrenaline flowing. It's calming because of the beauty of the natural environment. There is also a kindred spirit that exists among mountain bikers as they ride together. These elements combine to create active meditation at its best. To this day, I still get out on my mountain bike two or three days a week and enjoy time in the woods.

A few years ago, my brother inspired me to get a cross-country road bike. In nicer weather we ride for hours, getting lost in conversation and spending time together. We have participated in several century rides—riding across a hundred miles at a single clip. It is definitely hard work but very rewarding, especially when riding through beautiful scenery. While my brother and I are weekend warriors when it comes to biking, many people ride as their own personal escape from reality.

Eduardo Espitia is a certified public accountant in Briarcliff Manor, New York, and has been an avid cyclist for over twenty years. Eduardo started his cycling career in college and rode four times a week for an average of forty to sixty miles a ride. He was doing well, so a friend encouraged him to start racing, and he has been racing ever since. I met Eduardo when he enrolled his two children in my martial-arts school, and we started talking about bicycling. I was very impressed with his passion and the amount of riding and training he does.

Eduardo rides five or six days a week and races ten to fifteen times a year. He is part of a team of ten that trains, rides, and competes together throughout the Western Hemisphere. With Eduardo's extensive experience and passion, I wanted to get his take on how he sees riding as a form of meditation.

"Riding is all about being relaxed and controlling the breathing. When you do so, you become one with the bike," he explained.

Timing the inhale and exhale with the stroke of the pedals is key to riding efficiently. Efficiency is integral in riding long distances and racing because you have to reserve as much energy as possible. Frequent cyclists find that the more rhythmic they are with their breathing and pedaling, the more success they have. Shoes made specifically for cycling can also aid an efficient ride. When you get into the rhythmic motion of pedaling while aligned with proper breathing, meditative benefits come to the surface—you are able to lose yourself in the ride.

There are two types of meditation in cycling: hard-effort riding, which many cyclists call "high-zone" or "max-zone" riding; and easy-effort riding, or "low-zone" riding. Both parts have a meditative element, but with different approaches.

Hard-effort riding typically is necessary when climbing hills and pushing the heart rate up as high as it can go, putting forth maximum effort. When facing a high-effort challenge, Eduardo suggested choosing a word to repeat that empowers you. Eduardo's word is *power*. When I have an intense climb, I personally repeat the phrase "Yes, I can" as I face my uphill challenge. It doesn't matter what you say, as long as the mantra resonates with you and helps you push through the pain. The intensified mantra also exaggerates the inhale and exhale of breath, allowing you to continue breathing in alignment with your effort. Meditation comes to play in hard-effort riding through concentration—the body will insist on giving up, but the mind can overcome the resistance. Hard-effort riding is a strong form of performance-based meditation.

Easy-effort riding tends to be meditative in a different way—it gives you the opportunity to let your mind go. Easy-effort riding is a rejuvenation meditation, where you can lose yourself in the repetition of motion and let your mind wander. This not only allows your mind to rejuvenate, but also gives your body a break, especially if following a hard-effort ride.

Many elite racers believe in the power of visualization and

alternative styles of meditation, such as yoga and sitting meditation. This allows the athletes to remain calm before the intensity of a race. Eduardo was always amazed at how professional athletes can begin a race looking as calm as ever while also extending 100 percent effort.

Eduardo is part of a team and trains often with the friends he races with. They range from young adults to more seasoned adults with families. They all share the same passion for riding and racing. The comradery and support they develop in their training and racing help challenge and elevate each of them. In a team, the energy that would normally flow through you as an individual is combined with the energy of others and magnified as everyone works synergistically toward a common goal. This is the beauty of training with a team. You are all sharing in a meditative experience, where the cadence and rhythm of riding is the same throughout the group.

There are many safety precautions when it comes to riding. Most methods of active meditation are based on you, and not with a mechanical object such as a bicycle. You could travel far and be stranded if you do not prepare properly. Eduardo stressed that in order for you to take on riding as a form of your own meditation, you need to gain some specialized knowledge. This includes several factors.

Proper Nutrition: Nutrition and hydration are key elements. There is a term in the cycling world called "bonking," which refers to nutritional depletion and very low energy. The majority of the time, this is due to lack of nourishment. According to Eduardo, a specific nutrition plan should be followed before embarking on a ride, during the ride, and after the ride. It could make all the difference between an enjoyable or torturous experience. Many experts say that you should drink one bottle of water per hour to stay properly hydrated during a ride. You also need to replenish your electrolytes to be able to sustain your energy for extended rides.

Buy a Bike Properly Fitted for You: There is nothing like having good equipment, especially if you are going to ride regularly. Be sure to go to a local bike shop and get a bike that properly fits you. This will both ensure that you are comfortable on the ride as well as help reduce the possibility of injury.

Practicing Road Safety: Safety is key. Always remember to wear a helmet; no matter what kind of riding you do. Reaching a meditative state while riding is achievable, but cyclists cannot lose awareness of their surroundings, especially on the road with traffic. Always ride in the same direction as traffic, and be defensive at all times. If you are just starting out, research local bike paths and low-traffic areas where you can ride. Once you feel comfortable in the bike-only environment, then consider venturing off onto higher-traffic roads. Always have a spare tire tube with you, and have a cell phone with you in case of emergency. It is also a great idea to let someone know what path you plan on riding.

Bicycling is a wonderful method to achieve active meditation, and it can be extremely enjoyable for the whole family. It is a very healthful form of exercise that gets you outside, around nature, and with people you care about. Listen to your body and enjoy the ride. If you push your body beyond its capability, you will not have a positive experience. The meditative experience comes from feeling comfortable, allowing energy to flow freely, and being sure to go on rides that fit your capability and interests.

Action Steps to Begin Bicycling

1. Get a bicycle properly fitted.

2. Find a local bike path or low-traffic road where you can ride safely.

3. Always wear a helmet, and take all safety precautions.

4. Research what type of riding you would like to get involved in—mountain biking or road riding.

5. Take a clinic and get started before you venture out on your own, especially mountain biking.

Foster a Meditative Environment While Bicycling:

1. Relax. Be consciously aware of relaxing your muscles as you ride.

2. Time your breathing to match each pedal stroke. Create a comfortable cadence.

3. Create a mantra to overcome high-effort fatigue.

4. Be aware of your body, your environment, and the effort you are putting forth to create a meditative experience.

I hear the same advice from endurance swimmers, runners, bikers, walkers, and hikers: the most important thing is to just get out there solely for the enjoyment. Do that, and you will find yourself having a meditative experience. It is important to know that every activity has the opportunity to be challenging. If you are on an open swim, there may be tides or currents. For land activities, you will have to contend with both uphill and downhill terrain, but I've found that the variety always adds to the experience. One final note: embrace whatever you experience wholly, with one mind, free from distraction. If you feel and experience the different parts of your body and be mindful of your thoughts, feelings, actions, and the environment, then you will experience great meditative benefits.

....

Chapter 8 Key Points:

- A runner's high is a state of being in which one experiences running at a spiritual level with no physical exertion whatsoever.

- Mindful swimming requires the coordination of breath and stroke to the point where the swim becomes rhythmic and automatic.

- There are two types of meditation in cycling: hard-effort riding, which many cyclists call "high-zone" or "max-zone" riding; and easy-effort riding, or "low-zone" riding.

- Enjoying whichever physical activity you choose is the most efficient way to achieve active meditation.

....

Chapter 9

Being in Nature: Hiking, Gardening, and Landscaping

My spiritual journey was propelled forward when Grandmaster Kim invited all master instructors to visit a meditation master in Korea. It was an experience like no other, and it would be a book in itself to describe. In order to see the meditation master, we had to eat vegetarian, drink organic wild green tea, and practice sitting meditation daily. The meditation master also suggested we read *Living with the Himalayan Masters* by Swami Rama. I finished reading the book on the plane to Korea, and, to be honest, reading the book was a frustrating experience because I was relatively young and had really only done physical training up until that point.

Fast-forward ten years: I was cleaning out my closet because I was moving my family to a new house, and I found *Living with the Himalayan Masters* on the top shelf. I had tucked it away, not thinking I would ever read it again, but something triggered me to pick up the book and start reading again.

It was incredible! It was as if a lightbulb had gone off in my mind. It seemed that all of my physical, mental, and especially spiritual training had prepared me for the content in the book—as if all the mindful practices, meditation training, and personal-development training came together and made sense. I couldn't put the book down, because everything in it resonated with me. It is interesting what ten years of life experience can do for you.

When I had first read the book, I hadn't understood it at all, but ten years later, everything came into perspective. Every part of the book struck me to my core, especially the beginning, which discussed the importance of connecting with nature.

The following passage from *Living with the Himalayan Masters* describes what the author learned about the Himalayas, where he grew up. This is the exact reason why I spend so much time outdoors in nature.

> *The Himalayan sages taught me the gospel of nature. Then I started listening to the music coming from the blooming flowers, from the songs of the birds, and even from the smallest blade of grass and thorn of the bush. In everything lives the evidence of the beautiful. If one does not learn to listen to the music of nature and appreciate her beauty, then that which impels man to seek love at its fountain may be lost in the remotest antiquity. Do you need psychological analysis to discover in nature the source of so much happiness, of so many songs, dreams, and beauties?*

The gospel of nature speaks its parables from the glacial streams, the valleys laden with lilies, the forests covered with flowers, and the light of the stars. This gospel reveals the emphatic knowledge through which one learns truth and beholds the good in all its majesty and glory.

When one learns to hear the music of nature and appreciate her beauty, then his soul moves in harmony with its entire environment. His every movement and every sound will surely then find its due place in human society. The mind of man should be trained to love nature before he looks through the corridor of his life.

When one learns to appreciate fully the profundity of nature in its simplicity, then thoughts flow spontaneously in response to the appeals of his delicate senses when they come in contact with nature. This soul-vibrating experience, in its full harmony with the perfect orchestra of melodies and echoes, reflects from the sound of the ripples of the Ganges, the gushing of the winds, the rustling of the leaves and the roar of the thundering clouds. The light of the self is revealed and all the obstacles are removed. He ascends the top of the mountain, where he perceives the vast horizon. In the depth of silence is hidden the source of love. This music resounds in my ears and has become the song of my life.

The natural environment is beautiful beyond measure, and I find myself trying to "appreciate fully the profundity of nature" just about every day. I have been an avid outdoorsman and hiker for the majority of my life. I have hiked hundreds of miles on the Appalachian Trail and conquered many of the high peaks in the northeastern United States. I've met many people on the trail, but none are as passionate and knowledgeable about hiking as coach Mike Phipps. I met Coach Mike in 2012 when my wife and I joined the program Team in Training (TNT) to raise money for the Leukemia & Lymphoma Society (LLS). TNT has a great program—its members accomplish unbelievable endurance challenges while helping win the fight against blood cancers.

Mike was our TNT hike coach. We hiked all over the Hudson Valley in New York in the most amazing, remote areas I never knew about. But what made the training and experience so wonderful was Coach Mike's passion and knowledge about hiking. He had a connection with nature that I cannot even explain, and he inspires thousands of people to appreciate nature and all its wonders. He shares the same passion that Swami Rama describes in *Living with the Himalayan Masters*.

Coach Mike spends his days as an inspector for the New York City Police Department Housing Bureau, where he oversees all of the police officers patrolling the housing projects in the Bronx and Queens. Thousands of officers report to him regularly as they help maintain a peaceful, safe environment in the inner-city communities.

When I made a trip to the Bronx to visit him at his headquarters, he invited me to his office, which was decorated with awards, accolades, and pictures that represented all of his accomplishments in his thirty-five-plus years as a police officer. As we walked through the halls, his officers showed him genuine respect—that which only a true leader could command. He is a leader with a tremendous amount of responsibility, having to send his men and women into dangerous and potentially deadly situations. I don't know of a job with more pressure, yet he is as calm and cool as they come. Coach Mike and I went to lunch, where he told me about his passion for hiking and how it functions as a meditative activity that allows him to stay calm under pressure.

Coach Mike started hiking as a young child and spent most of his days exploring the outdoors. He only realized this was formally referred to as "hiking" when he became a Boy Scout leader. It didn't matter that Mike never knew hiking was the label for the activity he loved, because to Mike it was just something he did—he loved to be outside. Once he got hooked on hiking as an adult, Mike wanted all of the gadgets for the hobby. He couldn't get enough of the newest and greatest outdoor "stuff." This desire was magnified when he had a family and was able to take his own children to experience the outdoors.

In 2005, Coach Mike received a letter in the mail from LLS, which was looking for people interested in raising money by hiking the Grand Canyon. Mike immediately signed up and then had to figure out how to raise the $4,000 necessary to fund the hiking trip. In the beginning, it was all about the hike and not about the mission. As he made some phone calls, he heard heartbreaking stories of loved ones fighting the disease or who had lost the fight, and the donations just came flying in. It was then that Coach Mike realized the magnitude of the suffering that blood cancer causes. He told me, "When I tried to raise money, leukemia hit me in the face with friends and people I didn't know, and that put a reason to the mission."

By the following hiking season, Coach Mike had become the Local Chapter Coach for LLS, guiding and supporting people who wanted to help fundraise by hiking the Grand Canyon, the Rocky Mountains, and Yosemite National Park. Eventually, because of his accumulated knowledge of the outdoors as well as his great leadership and magnetic personality, TNT asked him to be the co-national team coach for the hiking program, and eventually he became the official national team hike coach. In this role, he trains and guides hundreds of people on endurance hikes in one of the major national parks.

When I asked Coach Mike why he has such a passion for the outdoors and hiking, he answered ". . . all the stresses in life—

especially being a cop—every stress starts inside the four walls of a building." He feels the majority of the pressures we experience in life are confined to the indoors, like career-based or financial stress. Being in nature gives us an opportunity to escape those stresses, if only temporarily. "All of the stress of the inside can be fixed by going outside," he added.

Many people who hike on a regular basis echo the same sentiment. When my brother and I backpacked on the Appalachian Trail, we would come back and express to each other how life is simpler on the trail. The biggest concerns in hiking have nothing to do with bills, responsibilities, jobs, kids, or anything other than physical concerns; the most important problem is finding your next water source or counting how many more miles between you and the next shelter or campsite.

As Kierkegaard once remarked: "To venture causes anxiety, but not to venture is to lose oneself. . . . And to venture to the highest sense is precisely to become conscious of one's self."

In other words, to "venture" and "become conscious of one's self" is akin to meditation, but how can *you* achieve active meditation on the trails? According to Coach Mike, "You have to have situational awareness and be present . . . [but] still be able to let your mind wander," he answered.

Because you are in a natural environment and away from your phone (hopefully), you get to be present in the moment and can let your thoughts wander. Author Tom Ryan describes the experience perfectly in his book, *Following Atticus*. For two years in a row, Ryan and his little dog Atticus attempted to hike all the four-thousand-foot peaks in New Hampshire twice in one winter. In the book, he writes, "I fell into a walking meditation of prayers, thoughts, and gratitude. It was so quiet, so still, so blissfully peaceful."

However, there are many hazards on the trail, so you must be aware even as you enjoy hiking as a form of meditation. You must always be careful on the trails because conditions could make what should be a very enjoyable experience a negative one. However, cognizance can actually add to the meditative experience rather than take away from it. The dual dynamic of necessary, heightened awareness and the relaxation of nature is an excellent way to quickly induce a meditative state.

How else can you encourage active meditation while hiking? During our interview, Coach Mike mentioned a technique called "tactical breathing"—also called deep breathing, discussed in Chapter 3 (page 21)—that can deepen your experience of meditation while hiking. "[Tactical breathing] also calms me down as I get to the hike. Sometimes when it is a challenging hike and I know it is coming, there is a nervousness that comes about and the deep breathing helps the nervousness subside," he explained.

Deep breathing during any outdoor activity is important; it maximizes the amount of oxygen in the bloodstream, providing increased energy, higher mental clarity, and amplified awareness.

Breathing in clean, fresh oxygen is a stimulating experience in and of itself. Deep (or tactical) breathing while hiking also allows you to monitor how you feel. For tips and breathing exercises, refer back to Chapter 3: Deep Breathing (page 21).

Coach Mike's advice for those who want to venture out into nature for a meditative experience is this: "You have to be safe. If you want meditation, start small. Always tell someone where you are, and have a plan to get back in case something goes wrong." It is also very smart to hike with a partner, rather than on your own. It's important to stay safe as you let your mind and body wander.

In *The Dharma Bums*, author Jack Kerouac describes hiking the mountains of Cascade National Park: "Try the meditation of the trail, just walk along looking at the trail at your feet and don't look about, and just fall into a trance as the ground zips by." This is the objective when it comes to walking, hiking, or just being in nature. To experience a connection with our natural environment is invigorating, to say the least. Accept, respect, and appreciate the natural beauty that surrounds you in nature. It is one of the most meditative experiences available.

Action Steps to Begin Hiking

1. Find a nice outdoor area where you can take an undisturbed walk—this could be in a local park, on a designated trail close to town, or in a heavily wooded area away from civilization.

2. Consider the length and difficulty level of your hike. Be sure to wear appropriate shoes and pack proper supplies, like clean socks, water, and high-protein snacks.

3. Find a buddy to hike with. If you would rather hike solo, be sure to tell someone where you are going. Use a trail register when available.

4. Take a trail map and keep emergency phone numbers with you. If there is no hardcopy of the trail map available, take a picture of the map at the trailhead.

5. Research meet-up hiking groups in your area—they're a great way to get introduced to local trails and hikers.

Foster a Meditative Environment While Hiking:

- Utilize all five senses. In addition to visually observing the beauty, breathe in fresh air through your nose, listen to the sounds, and rub your hands across trees and rocks.

- Relax. Be consciously aware of relaxing your muscles, especially your shoulders.

- Pause often. Allow yourself to appreciate your surroundings.

- Be aware of your body. Feel and experience the rhythm of each stride you take.

- Time your breathing with your steps. For example, inhale for three steps, and then exhale for three steps.

Gardening and Landscaping

Walking through the woods for hours on end may not appeal to everyone, but every person should experience time in nature.

Gardening and landscaping are pastimes that people all over the world have enjoyed for thousands of years. In the beginning, farming and harvesting were about survival. As time went on, gardening became an art itself. People found peace and tranquility when working with plant life. It is only since the advent of modern technology that society has become increasingly disconnected with nature. We were not born to be inside behind a desk and four walls all the time. As a species, we are hunters, gatherers, and harvesters who need to work with nature and be outdoors, whether by hiking, gardening, picnicking, or participating in sports.

Landscaping requires gardeners to work synergistically with the rules and laws of nature. As a gardener, you have to work diligently with natural forces much greater than you. Earth, sun, water, and air, along with a little seed, can create lush, beautiful gardens and an array of healthful foods. However, if you do not respect Mother Nature, she will take back what is hers.

The very first house that my wife and I purchased had once been held captive by nature. It stood abandoned for thirty years before my wife and I purchased it. To say it was a fixer-upper is an understatement. The property had beautiful potential, and since my father had a mechanical mind, he was able to look past the overgrowth and see beauty and master craftsmanship. It was a log cabin with exquisite stonework that emulated a castle. The house was in complete disarray when we found it—a tree was even growing through the living-room floor. My wife and I reclaimed the property and fixed it up into a beautiful house where we raised our family for over ten years.

Throughout that process, I learned that in order to work with nature, you have to consistently nurture the relationship through patience, diligence, and commitment—three qualities that are commonplace in gardening and landscaping. I had the opportunity to discuss gardening with two people who spend a great deal of time tending to their personal gardens. Patricia Santoro is a Bronx native and considers her gardening time her main stress-reliever. Gardening, she said, is her "vacation from everyday life."

Patricia compares her gardening experience to raising children. Children require a lot of nurturing and attention in order to become beautiful members of society. To Patricia, gardening is the same way. When you plant a seed, you need to nurture it, tend to it, provide the proper nutrients and water, provide adequate sunlight and shade, and work with nature to grow the seed into something beautiful.

During our interview, Patricia shared a saying that I often repeat to my martial-arts students: "What you put into it is what you'll get out of it." In other words, if you put forth the effort and diligence with the tending, your garden will flourish. If you neglect it, unwanted weeds will stifle the growth.

This idea relates not only to the tending of plant life, but also to

the tending of our bodies, minds, and souls. We are always planting seeds with our actions and thoughts in the hope that they will
produce the results we want. One of my favorite books, *As a Man
Thinketh* by James Allen, compares the mind to a garden:

> A man's mind may be likened to a garden, which may
> be intelligently cultivated or allowed to run wild; but
> whether cultivated or neglected, it must, and will,
> bring forth. If no useful seeds are put into it, then an
> abundance of useless weed seeds will fall therein, and
> will continue to produce their kind.

That is why Zen gardening has existed for thousands of years—
because of the ability to parallel one's life with the meaning and
representation of the garden. Zen gardening is mindfulness at its
best. When a person tends to their garden as an active form of
meditation, they are experiencing Zen gardening.

Among the benefits of mindful gardening is the ability to
engage with all of your senses. Hands-on work in the garden
helps strengthen the connection with nature—it allows you to
smell nature's aroma, touch the earth, interact with water, and
appreciate the sun, knowing that all of these elements will come
together to bring life forth from a little seed. Meditative gardening happens when you take the time to experience all of the elements of working with nature. It is empowering to think about,
and more so to experience. But most importantly: the results are
secondary to the process.

Patricia looks forward to working with the natural elements—earth, air, sun, and water. "It's simple, it's soothing. It's a vacation from daily life—away from the Internet, no music, no iPhone, no music. It's important to get back to nature."

Mark Nelson, a long-time Empowered Mastery client, has had a passion for his garden for many years. When we worked together, he mentioned time and time again how important gardening was for his physical and mental well-being. Mark shared that he experiences a meditative benefit at different stages of gardening. In the beginning, he walks his property and, he says, "dreams a little," visualizing what he would like to see in the year to come. During the growth period, Mark enjoys preparing his garden for new growth and watching every stage of progress. He anticipates seeing the fruits of his labor, predicting what the results may look like.

But more than anything else, Mark especially enjoys gardening because it is a joint effort with his wife. They both share in the passion and work together, which leads to a stronger relationship as they share the experience. They have many meaningful conversations working in their garden.

Therapists have come to realize that gardening and its meditative qualities can be wonderful therapy. Horticultural therapy, otherwise known as HT, utilizes garden therapies through working with plants and other elements of nature to improve social, spiritual, physical, and emotional well-being. Thousands of people have turned to garden therapies to help improve their self-image through the caring and nurturing of gardens and landscapes.

There are some things to watch out for that could hinder the meditative aspect of gardening. You want to stay away from "comparison gardening," or competing for a result, such as the biggest tomato, the largest flowerbed, or the greenest lawn. There is a different energy when you are building a garden for beauty, fresh fruits, and vegetables to feed your family, as opposed to building a garden as a competition. When competition comes to play, mindfulness is lost. Yes, you will get a great physical workout, but the meditative qualities do not come from an end product. The benefits of garden meditation and Zen gardening come from appreciating the process, spending time in nature, breathing fresh air, and working with natural elements to grow things of beauty.

Avoid using machinery during the gardening process unless absolutely necessary. Mark and Patricia both mentioned that the experience of hands-on gardening reinforces the connection between the gardener and the garden. When you add machinery into the mix, the connection becomes tainted and it creates a barrier between you and nature. Use hand tools, be willing to get your hands dirty, and utilize all of your senses when working in your garden.

For some, having an outdoor garden may not be feasible, but it is possible to experience the similar meditative benefits through indoor gardening. There is always the option to organize your own mini-greenhouse, place plant stands throughout your home, or utilize any open windowsills. If your space is especially small, you could grow succulents—very small plants that require lots of sunlight and little water. Many people who live in urban areas and cities have even ventured off to do gardening in the community through local garden clubs. If you are interested in exploring gardening as a form of meditation and don't know where to start, the best thing to do is search for a local gardening group. These groups have a wealth of knowledge to share, and they will be able to steer you in the right direction.

Action Steps to Begin Gardening as a Form of Meditation

1. Identify an area where you would like to start a garden—whether on your own property, in a community garden, or even in your house.

2. Map out your garden. Walk around existing gardens or do research online to get ideas about what you like.

3. Start small. Experience success and grow your garden from there.

4. Ask for help. Be sure to ask professionals for advice on where to get seeds and plants. Many have a wealth of knowledge and will be happy to help.

....

Foster a Meditative Environment While Gardening:

- Utilize your senses. Breathe in fresh air, smell the natural aromas, touch the dirt, and hear the sounds of nature.

- Disconnect; garden without your smartphone. Just be one with nature, free from distraction.

- Be mindful of your actions; gardening meditation lies in the process, not the end product.

- Stay away from machinery unless absolutely necessary. It may take longer, and that's okay—it will just give you more opportunity to be with your garden.

....

Chapter 10

Art and Creativity

A number of years ago, I was at a local health club with my family. While I was waiting in the lobby, I noticed some artwork that was for sale on the walls. One particular painting was of a beautiful horse. It was vibrant and powerful—a true work of art. I began to think about how awesome it would be to take the thoughts and images in my mind and depict them on canvas. I imagined painting martial-arts techniques and felt frustrated when I realized it was beyond my abilities. I decided to take an art class.

After searching for a local class, I found the Art Academy of Westchester and spoke to its founder, Vicente Saavedra. Vicente was extremely helpful, and, as it turned out, the school had exactly what I was looking for. My wife and I both signed up for their weekly beginner's class.

In the beginning, the class was humbling, to say the least. Coming from a family of artists, I half expected to be fairly artistic. I had a clear image in my mind of what I wanted to draw, but for some reason it rarely took form on paper. The fact is, I really wanted to paint, but I didn't have the abilities yet. After the first group of classes, I picked a sculpture to draw as my ongoing project. My sculpture was the head of a zebra, and my wife was drawing a statue of a stallion. I was immediately impressed by the level of attention and detail it took to represent the sculptures on even a basic level.

As I was working on my zebra, time just escaped me. My weekly allotted time to work on the project seemed to end as soon as it began. There were no cell phones, no distractions—just my easel, my paper, my pencil, my (frequently used) eraser, and myself. The instructor, Cami, would walk around and give subtle suggestions and constant positive encouragement, but never tried to alter the direction of the work. It was definitely one of the most meditative experiences of my life. I have always spent my time training physically, and this was the first time I'd participated in what I consider a "soft" activity. Ironically, there were times when I was totally exhausted after my class, as if I had participated in an endurance activity—all because I was mentally, spiritually, and physically invested in my artwork.

Vicente is a true artist to the core. His work is filled with emotion and passion that only an artist could explain. It is amazing how his pieces can tell a story with just a single pose.

Vicente began his art career at a very young age. He was born in Venezuela and moved to the United States when he was a small child. He remembers art being a constant part of his upbringing. During our interview, he explained that art was never something he had to think about; it was just something he did as if it were always a part of him. "Art was just about doing it . . . it was inside of me and very active in my family," he said.

It was around eighth grade that he began drawing pictures of Olympic athletes. Shortly after, he decided to become a little more serious about acquiring skill and began taking art classes in high school. Vicente admitted to me that he really didn't enjoy traditional school—all he wanted to do was paint and play music.

When it was time to go to school, his father encouraged him not to go for art but for something outside of his comfort zone. As Vicente explained, "My father said to go to school to get educated in something different than art, because [I would] always have art. So I didn't go to school to learn art but always had the passion."

Vicente took his father's advice and went to college to study political science. He graduated but continued to have a passion for the arts. Right out of college, Vicente went to work in the financial industry, but always felt there was a void in his life. "I honestly didn't enjoy the job and always wanted to transition to the arts; it was what I was meant to do. I knew I wanted to but didn't know how to make the switch from art to music," he said.

In 2008, Vicente finally realized his dream when he was let go from his job in the financial industry. It was then that he opened the Academy to teach art for a living. "People thought I was crazy, but I knew what I wanted and needed to do, and I know my teaching style works. I was confident," he explained.

Just like Vicente's assurance that he loves art because, as he says, "It was always a part of me," the practice of creating has always felt natural to him. The amount of focus necessary to translate thought to visual art can induce a meditative state as naturally as seated meditation. Vicente added, "For adults, it gets quite intense, because they are focusing on a single thing. The realization gained drawing from observation can be so challenging by itself. The connection between you and the task can be incredibly meditative."

He went on to say, "Building skills: creating, concentrating, solving mysteries of the mind, and getting lost in what they are doing. . . . What could be more mentally and spiritually rewarding than creating art? Feeling alive and doing something that only humans could do—it's as good as life gets."

Regarding his own work as a form of meditation, Vicente now blocks out time to paint once or twice a week on his own and can easily spend two to three hours at a time immersed in what he is doing. In fact, if he spends less time than that on his artwork, he feels like he can't lose himself completely, so he tries to avoid shorter sessions.

Vicente also has a passion for music that is as strong as his passion for art. Since he is sometimes too busy to block out the two or three hours for his painting, Vicente fills his artistic void by playing music. He plays the *guitarrón*, a large guitar with a deep powerful sound, and he also plays music in a French band that performs at local venues. Vicente plays music he conducted and covers popular French hits from the thirties to the seventies, including music from artists such as Jacques Brel, Édith Piaf, and Yves Montand. He says that his music becomes so meditative that many times he has even fallen asleep with the guitarrón on his lap.

Vicente looks at his music as another creative outlet and feels the same pleasure when losing himself in the creation of pictures or words. "Creative people are closer to God," he said. "There is a higher level of operation when the mind and heart are into doing. This is why I see my academy like my temple."

Vicente's paintings tell a variety of stories. One of his most expressive pieces features Medusa from Greek mythology. Most people know Medusa as evil, with hair made of venomous snakes and the ability to turn people to stone with just a look. Vicente created a painting to show Medusa as a creature of beauty instead of evil. "In my stories I try to bring the best out in people and elicit the beauty that everyone has. I look for the best of human conditions and show them. Everything is about creation. I always want to send a message that has a deeper meaning in both my art and music," he said. Telling stories and reinterpreting reality is another way to separate mind and body and allow enough space for peace and calm to enter your consciousness.

When Vicente is working on his paintings and other pieces of art, he shared that as much as painting could be relaxing and meditative, it can also be frustrating at times. Either way, it engulfs the mind, body, and spirit, and provides Vicente with an atmosphere of mindfulness where he is able to lose himself in his work.

"What is amazing is how the experience of painting can take my entire mind and spirit for many hours straight." To Vicente, art is a perfect avenue to escape life's challenges. "I am living the dream now," he said. "I got out of the finance industry and am able to teach and study art and language."

Whether or not you have a passion for music or art, you can still lose yourself in the focus and attention necessary to develop skill and create something beautiful.

Simple Mindful Activities

Even simple crafts can provide a great opportunity for active meditation. In Puerto Vallarta, Mexico, my wife goes to the beach to find seashells. She takes sand and shells from everywhere we vacation and collects them in hopes of someday making a glass-top coffee table with different sands from around the world.

She goes to the beach and finds a small piece of sea glass, then another and another. The corners are smooth and the fragments are rounded—they really are things of beauty. It takes hours to find the perfect pieces of glass. This activity—imagining and then identifying and collecting the most beautiful pieces of glass for her project—is a calm and peaceful, as well as absorbing, activity.

As a result, we now have a bunch of empty water bottles filled with the sea glass, and she's waiting for me to build her table. I look forward to spending my own meditative hours imagining and then constructing the perfect table to showcase what she's collected.

There are so many mindful activities that can serve as meditation—you never know what they might be until you experience them.

Coloring and Crafts

My daughter Stefanie is currently a student at the University of Vermont. With any college student, balancing school, work, friends, and being away from home are ever-present concerns. When Stefanie struggled with these problems, her adviser recommended that she pick up special coloring books designed for adults to help her when she is feeling anxious or overwhelmed with all of her responsibilities. The results have been remarkable. When she experiences any kind of stress or pressure, she goes to the library or her dorm room and spends time coloring.

In the January 2016 CNN article "Why adult coloring books are good for you," author Kelly Fitzpatrick states:

> According to the American Art Therapy Association, art therapy is a mental health method in which the process of making and creating artwork is used to "explore feelings, reconcile emotional conflicts, foster self-awareness, manage behavior and addictions, develop social skills, improve reality orientation, reduce anxiety, and increase self-esteem."

Coloring relaxes Stefanie tremendously, calms her mind, and provides her with the ability to cope with the challenges or situations that she faces.

"I think I like coloring so much because of how mindless it is for me to do. When I'm feeling stressed or anxious at any part of the day and I pick up my markers and start coloring, then the only thing my brain is thinking about is coloring in the lines of my picture," explained Stefanie. "My brain is somehow able to focus on only coloring in that moment and nothing else. So when I kind of need help getting myself calmed down, I know that coloring will be the only thing at the end of the day that will instantly make me feel better."

As I've mentioned, I come from an artistic family. My mother was a world-renowned cake decorator for many years. Her work was praised in *McCall's* magazine and routinely won first prize in major competitions. She made a number of amazing creations, including a gingerbread carnival, which included a carousel rotating on a large candy cane and a Ferris wheel. She did her work from 4:00 A.M. to 7:00 A.M., and I would always wake up to a house filled with the smell of fresh cakes and gingerbread. Clearly, she was able to find peace in her work when it was quiet and no one else was around. She found her own space even in a complicated life with a lot of responsibilities, and that's pretty remarkable. The greatest part is that she would always make some extra edible flowers (the roses were my favorite) or small gingerbread men for me.

I realize now that my mother spent a great deal of her life in active meditation mode. She was a pure artist and would often get lost in her creations. I remember she would always wake up early, have her coffee, and get her work done while everyone else was sleeping. During the day, she would manage the household as a single mother, taking care of four children as well as working to make enough money to support us all.

As she got older, she stopped decorating cakes and no longer made gingerbread houses, villages, or carnivals, but she found the same calm and peace by using her artistic tendencies to craft. She would continue to wake up at four o'clock in the morning, make her coffee, and get to work on her projects. She would take raw materials and turn them into pieces of art. She loved to create dolls out of crépe paper, design elegant wreaths, create needlepoint pieces, and much more. Her crafts were works of art with whatever she created, and each of my siblings still has her pieces in their homes.

My point is that most (if not all) of us have a pastime, hobby, or interest that we enjoy doing. It could be as simple as a cross-word puzzle or as involved as creating an artistic masterpiece like Vicente. It doesn't really matter what the activity is, as long as you are able to lose yourself in what you are doing. Be sure to block out time and allow yourself to have a mini-mental vaca-tion. If you have not found something that works for you, seek something out that will captivate your mind, relax your body, and release your spirit, and you will find a form of meditation that fits you.

If you haven't found a mindful activity that you identify with yet in this book, not to worry—there are more examples to come.

....

Chapter 10 Key Points:

- Artistic activities include a variety of hobbies— writing or playing music, sculpting, painting, or building, baking or decorating, etc.

- Art therapy—the process of making and creating artwork for healing purposes—fosters self-awareness, helps manage behavior and addictions, develops social skills, improves reality orientation, reduces anxiety, and increases self-esteem.

- Take advantage of classes and programs in your community if you're looking to get into an artistic activity.

- Work on your chosen artistic hobby (painting, sculpting, playing music) in a quiet place free from distraction.

....

Foster a Meditative Environment While Being Artistic:

- Don't just do the project, experience every aspect of your actions.

- Feel your tools. With painting and drawing, feel the brush against the canvas, pencil or charcoal against the paper and watch your creation come to life.

- Utilize solitude. Work in a quiet, distraction-free environment, with or without others.

- Prepare the environment. Meditation-style music and soft lighting will enhance the calming experience and allow the image in your head to transfer to your project more easily.

- Be patient. Pay attention to the details, no matter how minute; just appreciate the process and give yourself the gift of time.

Chapter 11

Moving Meditations

For thousands of years, people on the path to spiritual growth and enlightenment have engaged in a multitude of diverse spiritual practices. For instance, yoga dates back over 5,000 years and originates from northern India, but, according to a 2012 article from *Yoga Journal,* more than twenty million Americans currently consider themselves "yogis." Tai chi (pronounced "tie-chee") and qigong (pronounced "chee-kung") are ancient Chinese arts that also date back 5,000 years. An estimated three million people in the United States practice tai chi and qigong.

I still practice martial-arts training regularly, but over the past fifteen years I've shifted toward these less-intense elements of training. I have integrated the moving meditations of qigong, which are detailed in this chapter, into my traditional training to enable my development, both physically and spiritually.

Qigong

Through Japanese *ki* energy exercises (also known as *gi* in Korean culture and *qi* or *chi* in Chinese culture) taught by Grandmaster Kim, I have learned to increase my own personal energy while improving my flexibility and movements. *Ki*, *chi*, or *prana* refers to the life-giving force inherent in all living things. The exploration of ki has been prevalent for thousands of years. While tai chi and qigong have many similarities, there are many differences as well. By origin, tai chi is a martial art that integrates chi development through detailed movements against imaginary attackers—a common thread in most martial-arts training. Qigong is an art that explores the spread of your own chi to heal yourself or treat others. Qigong consists of shorter free-form motions that serve to isolate particular parts of the body and heal them. I am fortunate to have studied both in my training.

Both arts emphasize breathing in alignment with movement and the importance of relaxing the body to allow energy to flow freely. When the body tightens up, the energy will stop moving. Your body has to be relaxed to allow flow.

Sean Chillemi is a qigong instructor who has gained extensive experience in this field for the past ten years. At the age of twenty-one, Sean was diagnosed with malignant melanoma, a life-threatening skin cancer. He researched alternative treatments and discovered the Eastern healing art of qigong. He benefited so much from qigong that he healed his own cancer, and, as a result, he wanted to return the favor. Ever since, he has deeply immersed himself in studies and has committed his life to helping others. He estimated that in the past ten years, he has treated over 15,000 patients and helped them live healthier lives.

After spending some time with Sean, it was clear to me that he is extremely avid about his field of expertise. He shared some deep insights about qigong and tai chi and about why they are wonderful forms of meditation. Translated literally, *qi* means "life source" and *gong* means "the practice of"—combined, *qigong* translates to "life energy cultivation." Qigong is generally divided into two practices: waigong and neigong. Waigong is a physical outer practice, such as tai chi and bodily healing techniques. It is crucial to relax through every motion. During our interview, Sean reiterated to me (as Grandmaster Kim has mentioned many times) that the transfer of energy happens with the breath. Every time you inhale and exhale, you are moving chi throughout your body. This is the same with any movement meditation and the various methods of moving meditations described in this book.

Neigong is an internal practice that develops the inner, spiritual canvases of the body. In qigong training, neigong appears through specific motions that can trigger spontaneous movements of chi. For some, it is at that point that the energy seems to burst out. Waigong is designed to prepare you for neigong.

According to Sean, "[one] should be able to move like a wet

noodle to allow the flow of energy . . . and then have the force of a steel rod when needed. When you tighten up your body, your energy stops."

Both in tai chi and qigong, movements are generated to warm the joints, increase blood and lymphatic circulation, and increase oxygen so much that it changes the blood chemistry in the body. The theory is to utilize the flow of energy to heal yourself and others.

Sean recommended that anyone interested in exploring qigong or tai chi start with short forms of sitting meditation. He suggested sitting quietly and focusing solely on breathing, allowing thoughts to enter and leave the mind without paying particular attention to them. This is not a form of *active* meditation, but it is an important element of qigong.

Next, Sean recommended an exercise called the Buddhist Cycle. The Buddhist Cycle comprises the three-word chant, "omm, yenn, yah." The practitioner says these three words in succession for minutes at a time. The vibrations of sound throughout the body increase the energy flow to all internal organs, which leads to improved health. This is not necessarily a moving meditation but is accessible at any point in daily life.

Another simple yet powerful qigong exercise to increase personal energy involves saying the word "hong," spreading your arms as wide as possible, and completely relaxing the entire body. Envision the sun in the center of your body. As you breathe in, imagine you are stoking the flames of a fire. When you exhale and say "hong," it is as if a beam of light from the sun radiates out. Sean recommended that a beginner do this for five or ten minutes per day, once in the morning and once at night. This simple exercise will provide increased energy and improve your personal health and vitality.

When I asked Sean about the key element to know while enjoying these exercises, he replied "patience." Many people rush to feel better quickly, but they must realize that it takes time to reap benefits from anything. Many people damage their chi because of injury or sickness, so patience is essential to rebuild the body's meridians and build up internal energy.

Qigong healing is an art in which healing takes place through particular breathing and physical movements rather than physical medicine. The prescription? To practice moving meditation and free up any blockage of chi, and then increase energy flow to the injured area.

If you have the desire to increase your understanding of these exercises, seek out a qigong or tai chi instructor. Thousands of books and YouTube videos demonstrate various techniques; but to truly benefit from training, you should learn from a qualified instructor.

Bowing Meditation

Personally, one of my favorite forms of moving meditation (and one that I do in my own training) is bowing meditation. Bowing meditation is the simple act of performing a deep bow from a standing position, moving to a crouched position, and then back to standing. There are typically a certain number of deep bows that are completed in one exercise. The bowing technique has no religious meaning or significance; it is done purely for one's own spiritual and mental enhancement. Bowing meditation is a very beneficial and healthful exercise, but it is much more than *just* an exercise.

The essence of bowing meditation is humility and understanding that we are just a mere spot of existence in the world. Bowing meditation focuses on comprehending that we are beneath the universe, and on deepening respect for nature, people, animals, plants and all that is in existence. Bowing meditation humbles the soul and provides the ability to connect at a deeper level with your environment. At United Martial Arts Centers, the deep bow signifies a great level of respect. It's performed when our students receive their black belts at the tea ceremony.

Once an adult student commented that she was extremely uncomfortable performing a deep bow. She said, "I was told to never bow like that to anyone." I was definitely taken aback by that statement and explained the significance of the deep bow, how it represents humility and a deeper level of respect. I also explained that it's not only the students bowing to their instructors—I bow back. It demonstrates us showing respect to each other. The truth is that this particular student needed a little lesson in humility, and bowing meditation served her well. At the tea ceremony when the time came to accept her black belt, she did perform a deep bow, and all was fine.

There are many physical benefits to bowing meditation. Primarily, when you bow deeply, all the internal organs compress and decompress, which revitalizes them. The movement strengthens the leg and back muscles and improves flexibility throughout the whole body. There is a cardiovascular element to deep bowing as well, because it raises the heart rate and pumps more blood through the body, especially when done for an extended period. Deep breathing through the movement also oxygenates the bloodstream.

More significant than the physical benefits are the mental and spiritual benefits. Deep bowing increases internal energy through the act itself, the relaxation of the mind, and the alignment of breathing with the motion. Prolonged repetition of the bow allows one to lose him- or herself in the act, which heightens awareness of thoughts, feelings, emotions, and personal habits. This is an activity where the mind, body, and spirit work as one.

In the book *Zen Mind, Beginner's Mind: Informal Talks on Zen Meditation and Practice*, Japanese Zen Master Shunryu Suzuki shares his view on bowing meditation.

> By bowing, we are giving up ourselves to the universe.
> To give up ourselves means to give up our dualistic ideas

and become one. When you become one with everything
that exists, you find the true meaning of being.

Bowing meditation teaches humility and acceptance through
realizing that we are temporary guests of this world. Our material possessions do not really belong to us, but we have the gift
of using them during our existence. When we leave this earth,
we will take nothing with us, just as we bring nothing when we
are born. The simple act of deep bowing demonstrates that we
accept and respect the highest nature of existence.

How to Perform a Deep Bow

Just as with many art forms, there are variations of deep bowing.
I will share with you how Grandmaster Kim instructed me to
perform a deep bow.

To perform a deep bow, stand straight with your feet together
and with your palms pressed together in front of your heart.
Then squat down slowly and bend your knees fully, getting as
close to the ground as possible. Drop your knees to the floor and
shift off the balls of your feet so that the tops of your feet rest on
the floor as you shift your hips back over your heels. Bring your
torso down and compress your abdomen fully while running
your hands down the front of your legs to land in front of your
head, which should now be on or near the floor (this position is
similar to yoga's child's pose, but without extending the arms).
When your body is completely folded, raise your palms above

your head, facing upward. This action signifies a deeper level of respect and appreciation for life.

Now that the bow is completed, you will reverse the motion to a standing position. Raise your torso so you're sitting up straight, then shift the weight back onto the balls of your feet. Move back into a squatting position and stand. When you arrive at the standing position, open your arms as wide as you can and stretch them out fully, arching your back and tilting your head back as the arms come full circle to the starting point.

As you practice the motion, work to align your breathing so that, as you exhale, you are folding down into the deep bow position, and so the apex of the inhale coincides with your standing position. Remember, the inhale is bringing good, clean air into your system, and the exhale is ridding all the toxins from your body.

I personally perform 108 deep bows in my daily training. The number 108 is considered by many philosophies and religions throughout the world, including the dharmic religions and yoga, to be a sacred number. Mathematicians, astronomers, and scientists believe that 108 holds significance in their realms as well. I recommend that you research its meaning to determine whether that amount of deep bows makes sense to you. The other option is to block out a certain time frame (ten or fifteen minutes) to perform as many deep bows as you can.

A few years back, I set a personal goal to perform 108 deep bows every day for a year. I am happy to report that I was successful in doing this, although it was difficult at times. I remember being sick with the flu and fighting through my 108 bows, as well as having to complete 108 bows after climbing 8,000 feet in a single day. The funny thing is that no matter how I felt at the start of the exercise, I always felt better when I was done.

If you are looking for a simple form of moving meditation that will also provide health benefits, bowing meditation is a wonderful option. I also believe that many of us in this society could use lessons in humility, respect, and appreciation.

Yoga

Among the multitude of moving meditations, very few have the extensive worldwide popularity of yoga. Yoga has become a very common practice in American health clubs, recreational centers, and fitness studios. There are many different styles of yoga, and each emphasizes different elements of practice, such as flexibility, strengthening, meditation, awareness, spiritual growth, and even cleansing. In the United States, among the most popular kinds of yoga is hatha yoga—the foundation of all yoga styles. It embraces specific postures as well as regulated breathing and meditation to increase self-awareness. It is a holistic experience that serves as an excellent form of active meditation.

Michele Sardullo is a 200-hour certified yoga instructor who has been practicing yoga for over ten years. When Michele first started practicing yoga, it came easy for her, and she was good at it. Although she excelled physically, it wasn't until she started reading books on Buddhism and yoga that she realized its deeper purpose. She hadn't known about the spiritual element and went on a quest to learn more.

To further her knowledge and understanding of yoga, Michele spent three months living in a Buddhist community at a Tibetan temple in Northern California. She integrated herself into a community centralized on the concept of mindfulness and healthful living through sustaining a vegan diet and practicing Tibetan-style Kum Nye yoga. The key component of Kum Nye yoga is mindfulness and connecting inner and outer awareness.

Performing daily chores and tasks was required to live in the Buddhist community. Michele contributed by preparing sacred books to be shipped to Buddhist monks in Tibet. She spent all day wrapping the books in cloth and tying them, repeating the same tasks for hours on end with the goal of finding meaning in her actions. Michele found the repetitive work extremely calming and meditative. She also learned that practicing yoga was more of a lifestyle than an activity.

Michele shared a very powerful memory from her experience that expounded upon one of the deeper aspects of yoga.

> In my early twenties, I found myself in a Korean
> Buddhist temple in upstate New York. I sat in the

temple's meditation room, and a monk came to greet me. He was an American man, which was unusual in this community. I asked him how he found his way to live such a spiritual life, and he told me that his wife and child had died in a car accident that left him distraught and unable to cope with his pain. His friend, who was a monk, introduced him to meditation. He recalled that it was hard for him at first to sit with all those emotions that he buried for so long, but eventually he worked through it and found peace again. He explained that this [method is] referred to as "non-attachment."

I left the temple feeling very sad and confused and struggled with the idea that you should not attach yourself to people or feelings. I wanted nothing to do with meditation. I struggled with this conversation for a while until I eventually realized that what the monk was really telling me was not to be unattached, but to learn to accept. He was conveying that it was okay to feel hurt, pain, and sadness, and also to love, but to surrender the attachment.

As Michele learned during her stay at the Buddhist temple, the concept of non-attachment—stepping away from your own ego, beliefs, and feelings—is crucial for internal development. She explained that the essence of yoga is connecting your mind and body and preparing both for meditation. "The point of yoga is to prepare your body for meditation. Yoga is a moving meditation . . . which is why I really love to share it with other people. It makes you face yourself. When you find a pose that is difficult [for you] . . . that's the pose you need to do the most," she said.

This is very similar to many of the different styles of active meditation I've outlined in previous chapters. Being able to challenge yourself and develop mental fortitude is a way to higher self-awareness and understanding. This leads to self-confidence and will help you succeed in other areas of life. With yoga, it becomes a "calm confidence" in which the emphasis is relaxation and allowing the internal energy to flow freely and effortlessly, as in tai chi and qigong.

The main difference is that in yoga, poses are held for longer periods and breathing is aligned with the specific pose.

Inhale through the motion as you enter a pose, breathe deeply while holding the pose, and exhale through the motion as you exit the pose. When you exit one and enter another, you will breathe in alignment with whatever motion you do. The trick is to relax and allow the energy to flow freely as you transfer from pose to pose. The more you relax, the deeper the stretch will be. Some poses emphasize and focus on strengthening particular muscle groups; and by relaxing, you can isolate certain muscle groups.

As you are able to synchronize the movements with deep breathing, you will execute deeper poses with less effort. Yoga training will then become a viable form of active meditation, serving to develop your body through deep breathing, increased flexibility, lower blood pressure, looser hips, and improved posture. Mentally, yoga helps reduce stress, forces utilization of the diaphragm through deep breathing, and strengthens core muscles by practicing balance. Yoga also has spiritual benefits, although many yoga instructors choose not to push their students into that conversation.

"Yoga will help show [students] the path, but they have to realize it themselves," Michele explained. "Robert Ohotto, an intuitive life strategist, said, 'Others can only offer us the depth of intimacy that they have with themselves.'" In other words, yoga is not a practice that can be forced—it needs to be experienced. As the mind calms and and the level of internal awareness rises, you will find yourself appreciating and understanding the essence of yoga.

For beginners seeking out a yoga program, Michelle emphasized that it is crucial to have an open mind. Many advanced poses are intimidating for newcomers interested in getting started, so Michele recommends finding a likable, relatable, and knowledgeable teacher. Seek out local exercise centers, health clubs, boutiques, or recreational programs for a beginner's yoga program to get started. If practicing yoga resonates with you, pursue it at a deeper level. As with any new activity, patience is key—enjoy the process of *learning* yoga, not perfecting the practice.

Yoga is about internal growth and the relationship you have with your true self. In researching more of the essence of yoga,

I came across this description by Dr. Swami Shankardev Saraswati, published in an August 2007 article in *Yoga Journal*:

> Yoga . . . is any method that allows us to wake up to who we really are and to what life is all about. Anything that allows us to be more aware of ourselves and to feel connected to ourselves and life is a form of yoga. It could arise from having a cup of tea, as is done in Japan in formal tea ceremonies. Or it could be the sense of connection that comes from doing something you enjoy like sports or gardening. Everything we do can become yoga if it is done with awareness. . . .
>
> The key to yoga is awareness—discovering the luminous intelligence that lies within us all. When we find and cultivate this aspect of ourselves, we create our own health, happiness, and peace which we can then, in turn, convey to others.

Chapter 11 Key Points:

- **More than twenty million Americans practice yoga, and an estimated three million Americans practice tai chi and/or qigong.**

- **Moving meditations emphasize breathing in alignment with movement and the importance**

of relaxing the body to allow energy to flow
freely.

- If you wish to start up tai chi, qigong, or yoga,
  research programs in your community and
  learn from a licensed instructor.

- If you choose to practice bowing meditation,
  be sure to start by practicing deep bows for a
  short amount of time—ten or fifteen minutes,
  perhaps—and work your way up to 108 bows
  at a time or more.

- No matter which moving meditation you choose,
  breathing properly is much more important than
  perfecting the physical movement.

....

Foster a Meditative Environment While Practicing Moving Meditations:

- Breathe and relax. Remember, breathing is
  essential in moving internal energy through
  your body, and relaxing allows the energy to
  flow. Be aware of your breathing during all
  moving meditations.

- Stay mindful. This is the number one concept I recommend for anyone exploring meditative practices. Stay cognizant of the motions and work to breathe in conjunction with the movements.

- Practice regularly. Repetition is vital to understanding the exercises at a subconscious level. Practice develops muscle memory, which allows you to achieve a state of "being" instead of just "doing."

- Be creative, not competitive. Work hard to focus on your own individual progress and create an experience that is meaningful for yourself. Do not compete or compare with anyone else. That will defeat the purpose of moving meditation and mindful activities.

- Practice in nature. Many of my most memorable training experiences are outside in nature. The sounds of nature serve as a wonderful background for practicing techniques to the point that they become instinctive and natural.

Chapter 12

Martial Arts

I have dedicated the last thirty-plus years to the practice and expansion of martial arts and its values. On the surface, many people believe that martial arts is a fighting system designed for self-defense. And while it's true that a major component of martial arts is combat, to say that that is *all* it is severely underestimates the study's true meaning. The essence of martial-arts training is development of the body, mind, and spirit.

All martial arts have a physical component: a series of techniques designed to defend against attacks of all natures. My expertise is the Korean art of tae kwon do. In Korean, tae translates literally to "foot," kwon means "fist," and do translates to "the way of." So, tae kwon do is "the way of the foot and fist." When I first started my training, it was completely physical. I trained to win matches and worked tirelessly to become an Olympic-level athlete. After ten years of training vigorously and competing ferociously, I realized that tae kwon do was so much more than winning matches and tournaments. I searched to deepen my understanding of the art—it was all about the *do,* or "the way of," and a lot less about the foot and fist.

When I started training in 1983, tae kwon do was all physical. My original tae kwon do instructor, Grandmaster Robert Connolly, was a former heavyweight national champion and a fighter at his core. He trained us to win competitions, and that is exactly what we did. I, along with my training partners, Master Paul Melella and Master Joe Badini, focused our training on how to knock people out in the ring and how to win. We were specifically training for the 1988 Olympics, because that would be the first year that tae kwon do was an Olympic demonstration sport, which was the first step toward tae kwon do being recognized as an official Olympic sport, as it is today. We trained almost every day, up to two or three times per day. While we developed a wonderful set of skills and became elite competitors in the United States, we failed to make the US Olympic Team. However, after success in a variety of other venues—including a gold medal at the Junior Olympics and a bronze medal at the National Championships—I grew confident and developed an interest in teaching tae kwon do to others.

When I began teaching, I realized that martial-arts training is a lot more than scoring points and winning tournaments—it's a way of life. I finally began to focus on the *do*. This included learning how to help others benefit from the five tenets of tae kwon do: self-control, respect, indomitable spirit, integrity, and perseverance. I had the opportunity to teach children and adults how to apply these values to their training and personal lives, which was even more rewarding for me than training to win a championship.

After fifteen years with Grandmaster Robert Connolly, I was introduced to Grandmaster Kim. It was at this point that I learned the true essence of martial-arts training and realized that training is truly mind, body, and spirit. Grandmaster Kim believes that tae kwon do training is the answer to modern-day challenges, and that if more people practiced and trained, our world would be more peaceful. I have been following his guidance for over fifteen years now, and the training and development has been invaluable.

A Mastermind Meeting

Three times a year, the master instructor of UMAC hosts a weekend retreat that coincides with our black belt graduations. Students from all over the organization come together to bask in the martial-arts environment and develop their skills, foster their friendships and relationships, and develop physically, mentally, and spiritually. The weekend is packed with training to touch all aspects. Students are challenged physically as we push them to limits that they never thought they could achieve. Students are challenged mentally as they overcome the physical challenges they face. We also challenge them spiritually by waking them early in the morning to practice sitting and active styles of meditation.

When the training is done and the students have gone off to bed, the other master instructors and I debrief on the day's events and explore deeper and more meaningful conversations about martial arts—we call this the Mastermind Meeting. I took advantage of our latest retreat to ask how everyone views his or her own personal martial-arts training as a form of meditation. There were nine master instructors including myself in the room, ranging from fourth- to sixth-degree black belts, with anywhere from eighteen to over forty years of training. There were over 200 years of martial-arts experience in the room, and every master had dedicated his or her life to the practice and teaching of martial arts and the values that accompany it.

While some of us practice sitting meditation regularly and some not as often, every single one of the masters spoke of their training and teaching as their own sacred time. They may employ different forms of meditation for teaching and training, but they all consider their training as a time for reflection.

I found myself clarifying my definition of meditation at the very beginning of this discussion, however, because there were many misconceptions even in this group about what meditation is, exactly. Master Paul Edwards, for example, explained that he would become personally frustrated with sitting meditation because of its physical limitations. He explained that his muscles gets stiff in the standard sitting position, but when he adjusts, the meditation seems ruined. "I feel as if I'm not meditating correctly anymore," he said, then went on to describe how his thoughts are filled with "mind trash." Mind trash is negative, defeating thoughts. It's impossible to keep every one of our thousands of thoughts empowering and positive. Negative thoughts can fill up the mind and may even cloud judgment—this is mind trash.

However, despite struggling with mind trash during meditation, Master Melella explained that martial-arts training has the potential to remove negative thoughts. "Training is a whole mind/body connection, and when your endorphins kick in—sweating, working hard, and learning something new—that alone is a form of meditation. It gives you the ability to cleanse out all the negatives in your life—at least for the moment," he said.

During an interesting turn in the conversation, Master Edwards wondered whether meditation could be compared to Michael Jordan playing basketball and all his unbelievable achievements. Master Melella mentioned that Michael Jordan's coach, Phil Jackson, was actually a Zen master. He had his players practice meditation and visualization on a regular basis.

Master Melella himself often spends time in visualization meditation, picturing the goals he'd like to accomplish, like winning competitions, training, and growing his martial-arts school, and even building his own house. He relies on physical, mental, *and* spiritual training to accomplish his goals, from lifting weights or engaging in other meditative practices to visualizing the outcomes he would like to see.

Despite his regular training, Master Melella, along with Master Davin Sessa, noted that he doesn't practice meditation as often as he thinks he should. I took the opportunity to reiterate that both masters *have* been practicing, but in a non-traditional way. If they were training, they were meditating.

Martial-Arts Training as Meditation

Sensei Joe Joe, a veteran martial artist and martial-arts mentor I wrote about in Chapter 5: Mindfulness (page 39), was also at the Mastermind Meeting. He believes that teaching martial arts and training in martial arts are completely different—at least in terms of meditation.

"When I am training, it is meditation for sure. I look at the clock and see that I have an hour. Then I train, and [later] I look at the clock and notice that two hours [have] passed. I lose all concept of time. Doing without thinking is meditation to me. Knowing the purpose [of training] without having to reflect on it is also a form of meditation," he explained.

When he is fighting a competitor with an equal skill level, Sensei Joe Joe feels that he is absolutely in meditation mode—he can't think, only do. When in a dangerous situation, taking the time to contemplate each action rather than reacting on gut instinct could land you in trouble. When I spoke about this with Master Edwards during the Mastermind Meeting, he agreed and added that sparring is one of the most meditative experiences. In Chapter 2: What is Active Meditation? (page 12), I wrote about how Grandmaster Kim views sparring as a form of meditation and how this idea was life-changing for me.

During our conversation, Master Vinny Bellantoni shared that he views personal training as his form of meditation. When he's training and has a high level of determination and focused energy, he's not just going through the moves, but he's also becoming the vision that he has in his mind. If you were to ask Master Bellantoni "What are you thinking about during training?" his answer would always be the same: "What I could be doing better." This same determined mindset can be applied to other areas of life: work, home, play, or anything. "When I am training hard, I only focus on positive things and don't let negative things into my mind," said Master Bellantoni.

For Master Bellantoni and many other students of martial arts, learning certain techniques requires such concentration that it leaves no room for negative thinking. "There have been times when I have been training and my conscious mind wanders, and the mind trash sets back in," Master Bellantoni explained. "But when I am learning something new, I don't have room to think of anything else. Doing my personal best . . . definitely eliminates all of the negative voices that I sometimes face." If you struggle with mind trash when training alone, it may be beneficial to try group training. The experience can be similar to what Eduardo described about cycling in Chapter 8 (page 60). The synergy in the group is a total transfer of energy from one student or master to another, and everyone is working toward a common achievement. There exists the internal energy of not just one individual but a group working together, and it is nothing short of magical. Their physical techniques align with their breathing, creating a harmonious experience—as if they are all one, like a school of fish moving together in perfect synchrony.

Master Daniella Leifer had similar thoughts on group training but also on the concentration necessary to execute certain techniques—namely, *poomse* (also known as *forms*). Poomse are a series of blocks, strikes, and kicks meant to defend against multiple attackers.

"When I do poomse, I work to embrace the meaning of the form and invest myself into the pattern at an emotional level. . . . This kind of meditation fulfills me at a deeper level . . . where love, attention, and energy are used, which breeds creativity, and then that creativity breeds more creativity. It is when I am training that I get my deepest ideas," she explained.

At this point in the conversation, I chimed in and asked, "Are they deep ideas, or surface ideas like 'I need to go to the bank later'?"

Master Leifer answered, "Deeper ideas for sure, because the surface-level ideas are left as soon as I get on the mat."

I then addressed the entire group. "Has anyone ever trained and had something come up from the subconscious? Where you found a solution to a challenge, new idea, et cetera?"

Master Melella replied, "This just happened the other day. I was training in meditation, and a new design concept just came into my mind. I had to make a choice to either stop training and write it down or keep training and hope I remembered. I stopped, wrote it down, and kept on training. I couldn't or wouldn't have had that idea if I wasn't in a relaxed, meditative state."

Teaching Martial-Arts as Meditation

Everyone at our Mastermind Meeting is a professional martial artist who trains and teaches for a living. They all have active roles in their respective martial-arts schools and are intimately involved in working with the students.

At the beginning of the Mastermind Meeting, Sensei Joe Joe mentioned that teaching and training are very different aspects of martial arts. While everyone agreed, they also agreed that teaching students could also be considered a strong form of meditation. Sensei Joe Joe, Master Edwards, and Master Paul Maglietta continued with his perspective. The following is a transcript of our conversation:

> **Master Berlow:** Teaching is a form of meditation because you are the catalyst that brings everyone together to work toward the common goal.

Sensei Joe Joe: Teaching [is] also a form of meditation to an extent. Teaching is training as well, because I am ensuring that my technique is proper as I demonstrate. Whereas when I am training, I am not mindful of the technique and I just do [it] without thought.

Master Maglietta: Teaching is a form of meditation. I forget everything when I am teaching, because I work to manage all the students, instructors, and staff. I often get absorbed when all of us are working together with the common goal of helping the students be successful.

Master Edwards: When I am teaching, I am physically, mentally, and spiritually invested in my students, so I view that as a form of meditation as well—just [like when] I am cross-training and running, I am able to appreciate the beauty of the environment, and time and distance just fly by.

Master Berlow: Do you believe that when you are teaching you are doing a dual-part meditation, where both [you and the student] are working together syner-gistically toward a common goal?

Sensei Joe Joe: When I am teaching, I have to think to be able to help the student. Training is training, and teaching is teaching—you always have to train.

In the end, it became clear that a professional martial artist has to block out time for his or her own personal training as well as for teaching the students, as they really are two separate entities. I personally live by the rule that I have to earn the right to teach my students, and I do that by striving to improve my technique with my own training.

For many, martial-arts training is a necessity of our being. In other words, it becomes impossible to function if there is no opportunity to train. Master Sessa experienced this as he pursued a career in the financial services. Because of time constraints, he didn't have the opportunity to be involved in martial arts as much as he would have liked, and it became difficult for him to function. Without martial-arts training, which allowed him to focus completely and immerse himself in the pleasure of training and teaching, he was experiencing a void at a deep spiritual level. He explained: "As I am working right now and running my martial-arts school and I need it—I know that if I don't have my training, then the rest of my life is out of whack. I feel obligated to teach because I have met so many great people who have imparted their knowledge [to] me, [and] I want to do the same for others. I [have] a gift, and I want to spread it and help create a positive ripple."

Martial arts is a lot more than physical motions, it is a way of life—a lifestyle. Master Sessa works hard on teaching the philosophical aspects of martial arts as well as the physical training.

"Our culture focuses on the negative so much . . . [but] in martial arts, we get to home in on the progress made and not what's wrong," he continued. "[It's] a way that we can disassociate from the outside world and focus on our students' progress as well as our own. There is so much to be taught without actually having to physically teach it." Master Sessa then referenced *The Last Lecture*. Author Randy Pausch wrote this book for his children to demonstrate how the ability to show a positive attitude after being dealt a bad hand of cards, and making the best of it, can positively impact your life and the lives of those around you. In martial arts, this same perspective allows students and masters alike to teach and learn so many valuable characteristics, with one example being the five tenets of tae kwon do. We're able to both teach those values and apply them to our own lives all the time, to learn indirectly.

The Mastermind Meeting continued for three hours, until about 1:00 A.M. We continued to share our passions and perspectives on the profession that we all hold extremely close to our hearts. I truly believe we never have to work a day in our lives. In fact, I never say I have to go to work—I always say I have to go to the school. It is not work if you love what you do, and all of the men and women in that room are absolutely committed to the expansion of martial arts and its values.

Martial-arts training is the perfect venue to develop mindfulness. Its objective is to develop a state of mindfulness so that you may be consistently calm and centered.

As Master Leifer said, "Martial-arts training helps us find our better selves. [It's] an avenue for your own development, whether it be personal, professional, or spiritual."

You Know How Much You Know When You Realize How Much You Don't Know

After training in martial arts for over thirty years, I have come to many realizations. One example: we are always working toward self-mastery in our chosen field. For me, self-mastery comes through engaging in the mental and spiritual essence of tae kwon do. As time goes on, it shifts from less physical to more spiritual and mental training. A perfect example of this shift occurred in 2008 when I was in training for my sixth-degree black belt. Every day, Master Joe Badini would come to my house very early in the morning to practice for an hour, rain or shine, in preparation for the testing in Korea. We didn't miss a day, and we diligently practiced each of the techniques we knew we needed to perform. These are techniques that I have practiced for years, but during the course of this particular experience, something pretty amazing happened.

I developed a deeper understanding of the movements—more than I have ever experienced previously to the point that my mind-and-body connection was stronger than ever. During this training, I had a total, spiritual, out-of-body experience that I had never felt before. I was not "doing" the technique but rather "being" the technique. It was as if all the cells in my body worked together harmoniously to create magical movements with maximum power and precision. My breathing aligned with every motion, and the techniques were effortless. Here's the interesting part: the more I practiced and the higher the level I achieved, the more I realized how much room I still had to grow. When you deepen your level of understanding in a particular venue—whether it be in the martial arts, yoga, dance, or any individual-based activity—true growth is inevitable to the point that it is life-altering.

The beauty of martial arts training lies in the student. As I often explain to my students, like an artist expresses him- or herself on canvas, by use of a sculpting wheel, or on paper, if you are practicing martial arts, you are expressing yourself through your own body. Therefore, treat yourselves as your own masterpiece and pay attention to the intricate details of the technique. When you do so, you will experience the mind, body, and spirit connection that we continuously strive for.

Chapter 12 Key Points

If you want to get involved with martial arts:

1. Research martial-arts schools that emphasize the mental and spiritual elements of training as well as the physical. Interview potential schools and instructors, and be sure to be clear about what your objectives and goals are for training. Ask if their program can match your specific goals and objectives.

2. Take an evaluation or trial class to see if martial arts is the right fit for you.

3. Once you find a school, start training and embrace it with an open mind. You will do things that may be out of your comfort zone, but that is how true growth happens.

Foster a Meditative Environment While Training:

- Focus on progress, not perfection. This is the number one concept I recommend for anyone venturing into martial arts. There will be others who are stronger, faster, are more flexible, and have better coordination. As you train, focus on the progress you have made compared to when you started. This will help keep you inspired and confident as you move forward.

- Practice. What you put into your training is what you get out of it. When the instructor shows you techniques, you will retain the information better if you practice on your own. This will allow you to achieve a state of "being" instead of "doing."

- Patience is essential. The moves will not come easily, especially as you advance and learn techniques that are more difficult. Patience is the key. Always focus on the progress you have made.

- Be mindful of the environment. As an adult looking to engage in martial arts as a form of meditation, you will want to train with others who have the same interest. This will become evident quickly as you become engaged in classes.

- Practice in nature. Many of my most memorable training experiences have taken place outside in nature. The sounds of nature serve wonderfully as background noise for practicing your techniques to the point that they become instinctive and natural.

- Don't advance too quickly. Many martial arts schools will want you to test up to the next level quickly. Don't do it. Once you've learned the required motions necessary to test, add on an extra month of practice. This will help your motions originate from a subconscious level— a necessary place to be in order to perform masterfully.

Chapter 13

Dance

In my research for this book, I found myself thinking about all the different activities that allow people to achieve a meditative state. There are many activities that I have tried, but there are more that I have not had the opportunity to try. Dance is one of the latter. While I have always appreciated the beauty of dance and the passion of the dancers, I never made the connection until recently. My wife loves to go to functions where there is dancing, but I usually just watch her have a great time from the sidelines. When I do get the courage to jump in, I find myself going through my martial-arts techniques to the beat of the music. I prefer to stick to my martial-arts training! In my research, however, I found that dancing meditation is an actual practiced form of meditation that has been around for thousands of years in various cultures.

Dancing meditation involves letting go of all your inhibitions and allowing yourself to freely move in relation to the music. The goal is to get to a place where the body and mind are completely relaxed and experience the music with no constraints. It is amazing to watch dancers in action performing with incredible passion. I have often wondered how they are able to move with such grace and beauty, completely in sync with the music.

Fortunately, my martial-arts demonstration team was invited to perform at a fundraising event called Dancing for the Children, which featured a series of dance performances to raise money for a local children's center. Our demonstration was the first performance following intermission, so I had the opportunity to watch the first half of the show, and I was blown away. I was amazed at both the beauty of the motions and how the dancers were committed on an emotional level. There was a powerful story told through each number performed. I had to find out more about this art form, so I contacted the most well-known dance program in our community: Darcy's Academy of Dance and Performing Arts. Fortunately, Darcy's Academy happens to be run by my wife's childhood best friend, Darcy Baia-Cohen.

Darcy has been dancing since she was three years old, inspired by her mother, who was also a dancer. She was five years old when producers noticed her. After that, she started touring around the US with a dance academy. At the age of fifteen, she studied and performed in France and Switzerland. However, her true calling came at the age of nineteen, when she had an opportunity to teach. Although she loved to perform, teaching others was more meaningful and powerful. In 1993, she opened up Darcy's Academy of Dance and Performing Arts—it's now the premier dance studio in its community with countless national awards. Many of her students have gone on to study at The Juilliard School of dance, drama, and music in New York City.

When I asked Darcy why dancing was her passion, she said, "Dance is my therapy, my sanity. Nothing in life has touched me at such a deep level like I experience through dancing."

Over the years, as her school became more successful, Darcy found the ability to express her passion of dance through choreography. Darcy's performances are so powerful that many people have come up to her in tears because they became so emotionally connected with the performance. "Once I created a number and it was like I was letting go of something out of my own life. I tell stories through dance to uplift the human spirit," she said.

Darcy explained that dancing involves a constant and continuous state of meditation way before the performance begins. A great deal of visualization meditation goes into every number.

"Before I even [introduce] a new number to a group of dancers, I sit them down and have them visualize the meaning and purpose of the number, to experience the story they are going to portray. This gives them the ability to make an emotional connection between themselves and the story," she said.

Because of this exercise, the dancers' heads are at a different place when they are onstage. Darcy shared that some of her older students cry during more emotionally provocative numbers because the choreography touches them at such an emotional level. They completely disassociate their individual personalities and take on the persona required to elicit the meaning of the piece.

For beginners or experienced dancers looking to excel, breathing and relaxing are crucial. For breathing, it's recommended to inhale at the height of the stretch and exhale on the downward contraction, utilizing full range of motion within the movement. And the ability to relax is key to muscle manipulation and muscle memory. Dancers must relax in order to allow the energy to flow easily and effortlessly through them. When the body tightens up, the flow of energy stops and so does the dancer. When the energy flows and works in conjunction with the music, beauty through movement is achieved.

I asked Darcy her recommendation for beginners who wish to explore dancing: "Start in ballet because it is slow moving and there is a lot of work on the bar. You are able to focus on the technique of individual moves and don't need to worry about choreography. It is easy to apply proper breathing, and there is a lot of repetition involved. It helps to align the breathing with the technique, which prepares you to move with music."

Meditative experiences come to play when you are able to coordinate your body with music through routinely practicing choreography. Just like in any sport, repetitive practice creates muscle memory, and increased muscle memory requires less focus on the execution of a particular technique. With more practice comes more opportunity to focus on the choreography and emoting, and less on perfecting moves, which leads to active meditation. "At the point [of meditation], dancers could naturally let themselves go, and the mind connects synergistically with the music. Mind, body, and soul unite with the music."

Although this chapter has focused on professional and choreographed dance, dancing meditation doesn't need to take place in an academy. Many people choose to dance on their own, with their friends, or at social events. Whichever way it's done, dancing meditation provides a mental release and serves as a great form of meditation for a complete integration of mind, body, and spirit. The essence of dance meditation is to experience music through the body freely and effortlessly.

Chapter 13 Key Points

- To experience meditative dance, you have to lose yourself in the music. You will need to release any expectations and self-consciousness. This can be very difficult unless you are willing to let go of your own ego.

- Breathing and relaxing are of the utmost importance. Breathing moves energy through the body, and relaxing allows that energy to flow without constraint. Dancing meditation involves connecting the music with relaxed motion and engaging in breathing that coordinates with movement.

- Be mindful of the motions of your body and how they relate to the music. Start with slow, rhythmic music in order to familiarize yourself. When you feel comfortable, increase the speed of the music.

Chapter 14

Work

I have had numerous opportunities to travel to South Korea for training and touring the homeland of tae kwon do. Something I've noticed during my travels is the unique sense of personal pride that many Koreans seem to have in their livelihoods. Although many Americans put great stock in the fantastic work they do in the office, I have been repeatedly impressed by how many Korean workers fully embrace their trade as an extension of their personal and national pride. From the people operating the tollbooths to the sales clerks to executives, each takes a masterful approach to what they do.

On my first trip to South Korea in 2000, all of us masters were being fitted for *hanboks*—a traditional Korean suit to wear for formal occasions at martial-arts schools. The tailor didn't speak a word of English, but we learned that he was considered a master tailor in his culture. He took several measurements and some notes, and then he stared at each of us in turn for about ten seconds and wrote down some more notes. He looked at our skin tone, hair color, and eye color, and used the material that best matched our looks. We didn't have the opportunity to even choose a color; he chose for us—and did so perfectly. When we received the *hanboks* a few months later, the colors were perfectly suited for each of us. The tailor has dedicated his life to creating the best, highest-quality suits he can, and it was evident that he took great pride in his craft. Over ten years later, the suits still look as good as the day we received them.

In this chapter, we are going to meet some professionals who share the same level of pride in their work as the master tailor in Korea. There is a certain passion and love for what they do that allows them to "lose themselves" in their craft, and this in turn creates a meditative experience for themselves and sometimes others. For them, there is no "work" involved—it is pure love for what they do.

Meditation and the Massage Therapist

It is not hard to find a person who looks at his or her employment as a passion. You can do something as quotidian as filing papers or processing invoices and still accomplish these tasks with mindfulness. With enough attention given to the task at hand, you may find yourself effortlessly slipping into a meditation. That process amplifies when you care about the outcome of your work.

One person who feels that way is Laura Giacovas. Laura has

been a student of mine for over fifteen years and has achieved the prestigious rank of fifth-degree black belt in tae kwon do. She is also a master instructor. Laura is a wonderful case study of active meditation because all of her personal endeavors have steered her toward starting and operating her own wellness center in Westchester County, New York, called Soulauras Wellness Center. At Soulauras, Laura specializes in deep-tissue bodywork, therapeutic massage modalities—including deep-tissue acupressure, connective-tissue acupuncture, and shiatsu—and trigger-point myofascial release.

Laura began her career working in the children's special-education field. Her mission then was to help young children by creating a safe place for growth, learning, and sharing. During our interview, Laura noted that looking back, the special-education field in and of itself was extremely meditative. She worked with young children under five years old who had severe developmental delays. Because of her constancy, the children she taught could hold on to skills and achieve success in their later years.

However, the special-education career, as fulfilling as it was, was challenging all the same. Laura often felt overburdened and overwhelmed with the pressures and responsibilities of working with developmentally challenged kids, running a household, and caring for her own children. Eventually, Laura was able to find a comforting and supportive place for herself. "[Tae kwon do] was a clean slate and safe place for me to become who I was meant to be. It gave me the ability to reclaim my body, mind, and spirit. . . . Truly a gift," she said.

When I asked Laura how she looks at what she does at Sou-lauras as a form of meditation, her response was: "If you go with the premise that one of the purposes of meditation is to quiet the mind, still the body, and allow the awareness of spiritual connection, this is what I provide for the clients. In doing that, my work becomes beyond mental through the environment that has been created. The overriding theme for active meditation for me is gratitude. If I'm running, I am thinking for gratitude. When I am hands-on, holding acupressure points, and waiting for connective tissue release, I use a meditative breath and spell gratitude. Everything is meditative—when I drink my water in the morning, I spell gratitude. It's meditative because it is a sin-gular focus, can't think about anything else. I need to commu-nicate with life force energy (chi) so I need to be 100 percent present. The underlying philosophy is that when I am working on a client, 'I meet the body and greet the spirit,' as said by my bodywork mentor, Gail Kellstrom."

When I asked Laura to give a personal example of meditation at work, she described her sessions at Soulauras. To begin a ses-sion, she asks if there are any sensitive, painful areas. Through her years of meditative practice, she's come to believe that these painful spots are where the chi is likely to be blocked. She feels it is her job to open up the channels so the body can communicate freely, a task that puts her in a meditative state alongside the body she is working on. "If I could do deep-tissue acupressure on my clients while they are asleep," she said, "then we would be two people working as one in a state of meditation—I [would be] active and they [would be] deeply still."

The treatments that Laura performs on her clients, while extremely therapeutic, are often intense to the point clients could experience pain or discomfort. Many times, to get to the root of the problem, she has to work deep into the body. She has the ability to create an environment and experience where her clients receive the therapeutic benefits while they are in a sleep-like state and never experiencing any discomfort.

"When a client leaves Soulauras, I want them to have hope that things could be different, their body could be restored, that they could take ownership again and believe that they could do little things to enhance their quality of life," explained Laura. "They don't come to Soulauras for fuzzy slippers and a robe, they come to me because of serious injury, chronic pain, longstanding discomfort, and loss of quality of life. I do what I do to be a bringer of light and hope," she added.

To give some perspective on Laura's passion, she opened her practice, Soulauras, in 2011 after graduating from massage school. She opened Soulauras's doors two days later. Laura continues to teach tae kwon do at my center, runs Soulauras, and is currently back in school pursuing her third master's degree, learning acupuncture and Oriental medicine.

Laura spends the majority of her life in a state of active meditation through the combination of her profession and her daily practices. This is manifested in her constant reflection of gratitude throughout the day. It helps her focus and remain mindful even when she's performing mundane tasks that are integral to the success of her business and not necessarily what we'd think of as spiritual or meditative.

Meditation and the Professor

I recently had the opportunity to spend time with a New York University (NYU) Tisch School of the Arts professor, Nathan Flower. Nathan, who teaches classes in performing arts, sent me a YouTube video of his movement acting class. The students in the class were so engaged in what they were doing, it looked as if they weren't "doing" the activity, but rather "being" the activity. It was definitely a powerful form of meditation for the students; but surprisingly, Nathan related that it was for him as well. The experience of performing combined with the act of teaching is a passion that allows Nathan to access the mental state of active meditation.

Nathan realized his passion for drama as a college freshman at the University of Buffalo. He received a scholarship to UB for both his high academic marks and his love of the arts. He went on to receive a Master of Fine Arts degree from Rutgers University.

While in school, Nathan studied theater arts and frequently performed in community and regional theaters. He also spent time learning the technical aspects of performing arts by building sets. He started teaching in 1993 as part of a graduate fellowship on acting and movement and finished up with his MFA in 1997.

Nathan started down the path of fine arts because he loved the feeling of performance. Thanks to playing piano and percussion for over fifteen years, he feels very natural in front of an audience.

It wasn't until the middle of graduate school that Nathan discovered the deeper meaning of fine arts. He realized that his role was not to serve himself, but to serve others. An artist's job is to use their own art to affect people in a positive way, opening their minds and hearts to human stories that inspire change or even offer an escape from reality. It is magical when the audience understands the story behind the performance through the acting. In Nathan's words, "It's not about politics, sides of a spectrum, or religion—it's about the human behind the story. We have to remember that it is ultimately about the story of a human being. There is something powerful about a human story that opens hearts and minds and allows [people] to see through judgment."

Nathan feels that it is an amazing experience to see a crowd cheer for the villain because of the character's compelling back-

story. Through good acting, an audience can feel empathy—
even for a flawed character. An actor needs to be mentally and
spiritually invested in the role to perform at a level where he
or she can connect to the audience on an emotional level. This
cannot be done superficially and can only be achieved through
meditative practices. Removing one's own persona and taking on
another is a total immersion of mind, body, and spirit.

Drama can act as a form of meditation in two ways: during
training for the performance, and during the actual performance.

Training for the Performance

Actors practice meditation all the time in their training. To give
an example, Nathan shared a story about one of his mentors. He
explained how this mentor would start each class with a guided
meditation about letting go, being present in the moment, and
the current experience—a ten-minute exercise he called "ten minutes of nothing." The idea was to encourage the students to forget
about all their other circumstances for that moment. They would
also engage in movement after the meditation to get free from the
psychological noise—mind trash—in their heads. This gave them
the ability to start from a blank slate and experience the notion of
surrendering: letting go of the goal and the objective in order to
operate without ego, agenda, or the need to be "good."

To demonstrate one of the keys of being a successful actor or
performer, Nathan shared playwright Samuel Beckett's famous

quote: "Ever tried. Ever failed. No matter. Try again. Fail again. Fail better."

Nate elaborated by saying, "Actors need to balance their drive and desire with their willingness to fail, to risk, and stay open. . . . Acting is about taking risks—[you] have to be able to give up everything. . . . You have to find where your mind, body, [and] spirit work as one."

In order for an actor to reflect humanity back to the audience and do it well, she needs to first confront her own humanity—the good and the bad. If performers focus on their own opinions, they cannot take on the persona of another. According to Nathan, it is vital to "make the other people more important. Actors need to be totally present and aware. They need to work [from] moment to moment and be completely mindful."

Because it is such a competitive industry, it is important that aspiring actors have the mental fortitude to keep moving forward, so meditation can be quite important. Mediating the desire to be "good" with the pleasure that comes from acting can be difficult. Meditation helps keep actors and performers closer to their own center and mindful of their goals and objectives, so they are able to maintain their passion and remember why they entered the field of acting. Some performers like Nathan go on to teach the craft, and he shared that teaching can include some of the same struggles—as well as the benefits—of performing.

Nathan believes that teaching is comparable to acting in that you have to be completely present and engaged. You cannot think about anything else when you have a group in front of you. Many times it is as if you *are* acting when you are teaching, because you cannot bring your personal life into the classroom. The most rewarding teaching experience is when teaching becomes effortless with synergy between the instructor and the student; when there is an unexplainable connection and everyone feels they are working as one. There are times when an instructor will end a class and realize that it was extremely easy, fun, and productive.

Teaching is nothing more than the transfer of energy from the teacher to the students, which is the same as an actor to an audience. When two participants are on the same wavelength, magic happens. This magic is similar to an out-of-body experience, where one sees things from a third-person perspective. This is what I would call a spiritual experience or, as they say in professional sports, getting "in the zone." This can only be achieved through an enhanced state of mindfulness, being present, and, ultimately, through active meditation.

Performance

Performing is a form of meditation because when you practice so hard and so much, the performance becomes effortless. There is a degree of surrender involved. Nathan used the term "actor's faith," which refers to the commitment in what the actor believes in on stage. Actors question themselves as to where they are willing to go emotionally, imaginatively, psychologically, and physically to get the message across to the audience. "If you don't believe it, the audience won't believe it," Nathan shared. The same applies whether you are in front of a crowd, students, or an audience.

I always tell students in training to become instructors that children are like dogs. It sounds silly, but it's true. Children have the ability to read energy in the same way a dog has the ability to judge whether a stranger is a dog lover or not. If you are teaching children, and you are not passionate about what you are teaching, they will see right through the act and react accordingly. The same logic applies to the way Nathan explained actors performing in front of an audience. You, as the actor, have to believe, and when you surrender yourself to the role, you experience a wonderful state of meditation—you have completely let go of reality in order to fulfill the role of the performance.

"Surrendering and letting go of goals is key. Trust that you have done everything you need to do, and go with it. Just let it go, because you certainly can't force it or push through it," suggested Nathan.

Nathan and Laura are two people who have been able to find passion and meditation in their work. That is not always the case. My brother John, for example, is a lieutenant and paramedic for the local fire department in our community. I asked him if he sees any elements of his career as meditative. He gave it a lot of thought before answering "no." I challenged him and asked him to explain what happens and how he feels on an emergency call. He explained that it's as if time doesn't exist, and he is totally immersed in what he is doing. The only important thing at that time is to tend to the emergency—nothing else matters. I explained that he had just described active meditation, where mind, body, and spirit are engaged in a single activity. He agreed, but shared that emergency calls are definitely not relaxing. He's right—active meditation is not always relaxing; it can be quite vigorous at times, but it is always engaging.

Meditation and the Active Mind

There are so many different types of work scenarios and professions that are far from meditative, but not everything needs to be meditative. You don't *need* to love what you do to experience meditative benefits. It's not *what* you do but *how* you do it that changes any job or profession. This brings me back to Chapter 4: We Need to *Calm* Down, Not *Slow* Down (see page 27) and the concept of mindfulness. While at work, it's possible to achieve a meditative state, regardless of what you are doing, as long as you are being mindful.

It's possible to train yourself to be present by controlling your thoughts. This is extremely difficult now more than ever, with the influx of technology and interruptions that are common in the workplace these days. I have had clients create affirmations such as "I am present and mindful of my actions" to repeat during the day to help them maintain a present state of mind. For many of the clients I work with interested in improving their productivity, I recommend they go to a quiet office or library, turn off their phones and computers, step away from social media, and create an environment completely free from distraction. This fosters more productivity in a shorter amount of time.

In a world where it is extremely difficult to stay focused, no one needs a form of active meditation more than someone living with Attention Deficit Hyperactivity Disorder (ADHD). ADHD tendencies are defined by three separate core symptoms: inattention, hyperactivity, and impulsivity. Inattention causes those suffering from ADHD to become easily distracted; hyperactivity is the inability to stay still; and impulsivity refers to saying or doing things without thinking first.

Although many people experience some symptoms of ADHD, for those who have been diagnosed and live with it throughout their everyday lives, these symptoms are major lifestyle issues. Active meditation can be a crucial mechanism for mitigating the effects, with or without other treatment. I spoke to one of my clients, David A. Greenwood, who wrote *Overcoming Distractions: Thriving with Adult ADD/ADHD*, about how certain people utilize their ADHD to their advantage and have achieved high levels of success by doing so.

David himself was diagnosed with ADHD as a child and still has it today. As with anyone who has achieved success, David learned how to cope with his issues and even uses them as strengths in his life. He attributes his success to sticking to routines. In fact, David mentioned during our conversation that the routines themselves become somewhat meditative, because he is able to do them without thought—almost a kind of "effortless effort" as he moves through his daily responsibilities.

David also noted that as important as his routines are to help him stay focused and on task, it is extremely challenging for him to get back on track when the routine is interrupted. Enter the beauty of the ADHD mind. When David becomes hyper-focused on a project, he could easily knock out eight to ten hours of work and not even take a break or stop for lunch.

This doesn't always come easily. In fact, David needs to settle himself in for a bit before he is able to get into what he calls "focus mode." When he gets into this state, great things happen, and David experiences a form of meditation free of distraction from anyone and anything, but it requires preparation. To start, David arrives at his office and shuts everything down for about fifteen minutes so he can collect himself before he begins his day. "Getting in the zone and setting the brain on a certain mindset for the day [is necessary]. When you are hyper-focused, nothing else in the world matters," he said.

David also finds solitude by walking a three-mile path around a lake in his local community. He finds that when he is unable to focus at the office, he takes a walk in the woods to decompress and clear his mind before heading home.

"I'm not one to sit in a room and meditate—I can't sit still. Can I meditate while walking around the lake with the sounds of birds and wind? Absolutely," he explained.

One of the case studies in David's book follows a gentleman named Peter Shankman. Peter has achieved tremendous success in his life. He is the author of multiple books, including his latest, *Zombie Loyalists: Using Great Service to Create Rabid Fans*. He founded, operated, and sold a hugely successful company called Help A Reporter Out (HARO), a networking site that connects reporters with experts and sources for their stories. He is involved in multiple companies, is very active on social media, and travels around the world speaking on digital marketing, customer service, and ADHD.

I was able to hear Peter speak at a conference recently, and I was very impressed by both his message and his success. At the conference, he spoke about what he does to get "in the zone," and it involves highly intense active meditation. He finds that he is able to get in the zone when he is doing ultra-endurance training for an Ironman Triathlon or during the extreme activity of jumping out of an airplane. Yes, you heard it right: he gets his best ideas when he's jumping out of airplanes. These activities help his mind relax so he can let his thoughts flow freely.

Peter feels that when he is on a plane, he is able to focus on whatever he wants at that time. Because he is always traveling and speaking, he spends a great deal of time in the air. In 2014 alone he traveled over 250,000 miles. He wrote the first five chapters of his book *Zombie Loyalists* on a flight to Tokyo and the rest on the way back. For him, flying triggers some of his best ideas.

David is the same way. When he was writing his book, he rented a hotel room sixty miles away from his house. He would lock himself in the room, buckle down, and just write. He didn't stay at a local hotel, because he would be more inclined to meet someone for dinner and wouldn't be as productive. The beauty of being in the hotel room for David—or on an airplane for Peter—is that both these places encouraged a complete removal of distractions, which allowed the mind, body, and spirit to be completely present.

Peter has learned how to manage his ADHD by learning and understanding active ways to control and manage his mind. When I asked him what he does to calm down, his answer was that he doesn't calm down. Sometimes he looks at pictures before he goes to bed and that will put him to sleep; but for the most part, he is either in turbo-action mode or a mode of calm existence. He needs endorphins releasing into his system to make him feel alive.

When Peter comes home at night, he will stop at the front door, take ten deep breaths to calm his mind, and repeat the word "chill" before he goes in and sees his wife.

When I asked Peter how he views what he does as a form of meditation, he explained, "When I am in my happy place, I am able to manage anything. My meditation comes when I am doing things to allow my brain to reset."

During my interviews with both David and Peter, it became evident that both of them spend a great deal of time preparing for productivity. In other words, they time-block to prepare for active meditation. For Peter, this involves making sure he sets time aside for the activities that bring him the rush of endorphins he needs. For David, it's about taking the time to calm his mind so he is able to focus and be productive. This is why activities that engulf the mind, body, and spirit are so essential to all of us, especially if you have an ADHD mind.

Many people have a difficult time separating their work lives from their home lives. David has figured a way to quiet his mind before heading home so he can be more present and mentally available for his family. David brings up a key point here. Yes, when you get into the zone at work, it can be a form of active meditation. However, sometimes it may be difficult to switch gears, so it is important to take time for yourself to recharge your own batteries like David does.

We all spend a great deal of time at work—the average American adult works forty-seven-plus hours a week; and if you are an entrepreneur or a business owner, work typically begins when you open your eyes in the morning and ends when you close your eyes at night. With the need to spend so much time at work to uphold certain standards of living, you might as well enjoy it along the way. It all comes down to *how* you do your work and not *what* you do. If you take pride in what you do and have a positive attitude, any work will be a positive experience. Add mindfulness to the equation, and there's potential to experience the same meditative benefits as any hobby or interest you truly enjoy.

Chapter 14 Key Points:

- It is not *what* you are doing that determines whether an experience will be meditative, but *how* you do it. If you are mindful and aware, reaching a meditative state is possible.

- Schedule your time efficiently. Block out time to be as productive as possible. Set aside time for the activities that allow you to embrace your mind, body, and spirit.

- Allocate time for rejuvenation outside of work. If you are unable to create a meditative environment at work, then explore time to do so when you are not working. For some, this means taking a walk at lunch. For others, it means doing something enjoyable before or after work. Regardless of the activity, set time aside for yourself so you will be more productive.

Chapter 15

Parenthood

There are many parents who juggle multiple facets of life and don't have time to practice any form of meditation let alone do anything for themselves. Many parents in today's modern world have taken on the responsibility of working to supplement their income because of the rising cost of living in the United States. Their time is split among working raising a family, and managing a household. Many working parents have to make great sacrifices and find it hard to discover an outlet because they are being pulled—sometimes literally—in so many different directions. They want to spend time with their children but need to work to support the household, or they need to do the housework in order to free up time for something else. It becomes a constant "I need to get _____ done so I have time to do _____ . . ."—it becomes an endless cycle.

No matter how good you are at managing responsibilities, it's only possible to sustain the juggling act for so long. When you are a working parent and lead a chaotic life, you *need* to find some form of meditation that works for you.

Tricia Swatko is a working mom who manages her own career while maintaining a household and raising three children, one of whom has special needs. And somehow, she finds time for herself. How? Her method of managing all her commitments and saving time for meditation is incredibly impressive.

Tricia has been a graphic designer since she graduated from college. Before she had children, she worked for various magazines and scholastic journals; but after she had her first daughter, she quickly realized working fulltime wasn't a viable lifestyle for her. She decided to work from home as an independent contractor to spend more time with her child and minimize the amount of traveling and stress that comes from working in an office. She was able to maintain her business relationships and, without the need to search for work, she was able to maintain her career.

Tricia considers her job a passion. "I love what I do because it is a constant challenge to fix a problem. I get a feel-good high knowing I met the challenge, no matter what the challenge is," she explained. "I am always asking myself, 'How do I make [my work] stand out?'"

Tricia admitted that sometimes it's difficult to get into a meditative state—after all, she's a mom being pulled in a million different directions. "Sometimes there are too many thoughts, ideas, and things going on that cloud my mind. I have learned to cope with the challenges, so at times, right before bed, I will meditate on the challenge, and then [I will] wake up with the right solution." She relies on her career and her hobbies—planting and painting—to provide outlets for her energies and frustrations so that she can reach a place of clarity and retain balance in her life. Like my own mother, who balanced so much and would begin working at 4:00 A.M., Tricia had to find time to work.

"Sometimes late at night I get a bunch of work done while everyone is sleeping. When my children were younger, that was the best time to work. It became incredibly important, because my work was the only personal time I had for three main reasons: (1) I looked forward to it and got lost in it; (2) I was able to make it 'me time' without my children; and (3) I didn't lose who I was to just be Mommy," she said. It all comes down to balancing the areas of life that are most important to you.

Many professional parents out there work so they don't lose their identities and become just "Mommy" or "Daddy." Of course, there are few greater rewards in life than parenting and watching your children grow into successful members of society; however, what happens after they leave home and you don't have another outlet? The transition that occurs after children grow up and move away from home can leave many parents questioning their personal identity, because they may have lost sight of it after devoting themselves to raising children for so long. Sometimes moms and dads struggle to find themselves in the years between their own children's adulthoods and the time grandchildren are born. This is why everyone needs something to do outside their families, whether it be work or a hobby such as crafts, fitness, or sports. There just has to be something to fill once-busy time and make the transition to an empty nest easier.

But before the nest empties, it's important to find a way to fully engage with family while maintaining mental clarity—this is key for effective parenting. In this day and age, with portable technology, it's becoming increasingly difficult to be present with your children. Finding activities you can do together *without* technology will help strengthen your relationship with your children while providing, at times, a meditative atmosphere. This can be as simple as playing games with your children. If the parent is completely engaged in the activity with the child, then they are in a "zone" together. If you are able to balance time for your career, your children, and your own form of active meditation, you will be truly fulfilled in life.

The definition of sacrifice is the giving up of a lesser-value thing for the sake of something greater. This is exactly why Tricia decided to begin a home business rather than work a corporate job. Many moms and dads get this backward—they sacrifice quality time with their family for the sake of their work. At the end of life, most people never wish they had spent more time at the office. People usually wish they'd spent more time with loved ones. If you're a parent, you need to create an environment where you and your child/children can create memorable moments together through activities that you both enjoy. When time is shared between you and your children, you will experience a high form of meditation and give your children a lasting memory.

Many parents have a hard time turning their phones off during family time—they are often partially engaged but still connected to work or social media. Since part of meditation requires being present and in the moment, it is impossible to be completely engaged and mindful with such distractions. Meditation in any relationship comes from complete engagement with the other party. Nothing less will allow true, shared meditation with loved ones. When you are with your children, spouse, or loved ones, give them the gift of your time and energy, and be 100 percent present. I guarantee you will create memories that will last a lifetime for all involved.

One year, I had the perfect Father's Day. I woke up early and went on a mountain-bike ride with my friends, and then I spent the rest of the day with my family on a hike. Of course, the ride was great, but the hike was memorable. We had no technology; we just shared time with each other. The discussions we had were meaningful and enjoyable and, most importantly, positive. When the busyness and stress of life sets in, tempers can flare and relationships can become strained. Not on that day—it was all love, respect, and appreciation.

Parents, if you would like to create memorable moments with your children, ditch the technology. Make a point to engage completely and block out time in your schedule to do activities with your children, just as if you were setting up an appointment for work. Take them hiking or on a bike ride. Take them out for ice cream, throw a ball around, play a board game. To be honest, it doesn't matter what you do, as long as you spend the time mindfully. Master Melella said it best in a seminar: "We should treat our clients like our family and our family like our clients."

Chapter 15 Key Points

- Parents, in order to create memorable moments with your children, you will have to disconnect. As much as posting pictures to social media and letting the world know what is happening is important, it is not worth the expense of the moment.

- Despite your busy lifestyle, do your best to set aside time with your children. For example, hiking is a great activity that will keep everyone engaged and present.

- Parenting can be meditative as long as it is done mindfully. There are many stages in a child's development, and time goes by extremely fast. The more mindful you are, the more you will be able to capture experiences and positive memories that will last a lifetime.

Chapter 16

A Mindful Lifestyle

It doesn't really matter what you are doing, as long as you do it mindfully. As long as you can find the time to perform activities with intention, you will experience an opportunity to achieve active meditation. On page 46, I shared an essay I once wrote about time. For me, time is of the utmost importance, and I work hard to maximize my time and get the most out of my day. I strategically block out time for the activities that I enjoy so I can routinely experience the benefits of meditation both actively and inactively.

My wife also finds time to do activities she loves—activities that have become meditation for her. For example, she thoroughly enjoys cooking and preparing food. Ollie Nolan, her toy poodle, is also the frequent focus of her attention. She finds complete joy and relaxation in snuggling with Ollie as she reads or watches television. For her, caring for Ollie—taking him for walks, cooking for him, playing with him, and even cleaning up after him—is a form of active meditation, but minding an animal may not be meditative for everyone. When it comes to meditation, to each his own.

Throughout the day, we are involved in various tasks and activities related to our personal and professional lives. From the minute you wake up in the morning until you go to bed, you are engaged. Many people wake up and make themselves a cup of coffee. Someone living a mindful lifestyle will be fully aware of the process of making the coffee and utilize his or her five senses throughout the process. A mindful person will savor each sip, appreciate the smell, and be mindful of the action of drinking the coffee.

A mindful person will be aware of every aspect of his or her day. He will get ready for the day, fully aware of his actions and the sensations those actions present. When in conversation, his mind is completely focused. Mindfulness comes when one lives in the moment and appreciates the act of *doing* rather than just striving to achieve an outcome.

A good place to start practicing mindfulness is at the dinner table. America has become a fast-food nation, but the very idea of fast food contradicts everything that mindfulness tries to achieve. When you eat, there is a delay between your mind and your stomach. It takes time for the brain to comprehend that the stomach is full. When children and adults eat too quickly, they end up overeating, because the brain doesn't have time to register that the stomach is full.

Mindful eating habits enable people to not only appreciate their food more, but also allow the brain time to process that it has eaten—in this way, mindfulness at the dinner table can benefit health. To achieve mindful eating, sit at a table and take one spoonful or forkful of food at a time, making sure to set down your utensil between each bite. Savor the flavors and textures of your meal, and take the time to chew thoroughly before swallowing.

When it comes to your career, focus more on the act of doing and be aware of the process, rather than just working so you can finish.

I have tried to share a similar strategy with my children. They tend to take a very long time to finish their schoolwork because music is on, phones are by their sides, social-media feeds are in front of them, and distractions are all over. I explain to them exactly what I explain to my clients: focus on what you *need* to do, and lose all the stuff that brings you distraction—you'll finish your work in half the time. You will then have more time to do what you want. The alternative is to spend twice the time getting half the work done and still have more to do later. It doesn't make sense.

The point is, any hobby or interest that you engage in could easily be a form of active meditation depending on how you, the aspirant, approach it. Many people find their own escape from reality through gardening, horseback riding, kayaking, rock climbing, pottery, music, backpacking, jewelry making, glass blowing, wine making, beer brewing, geocaching, rock collecting, drawing, and more. The only crucial element is that whatever you choose to do or engage in should be something that will allow the integration of mind, body, and spirit to focus on one thing. Mindful living means taking even the mundane life activities as well as your hobbies and turning them into mindful meditation.

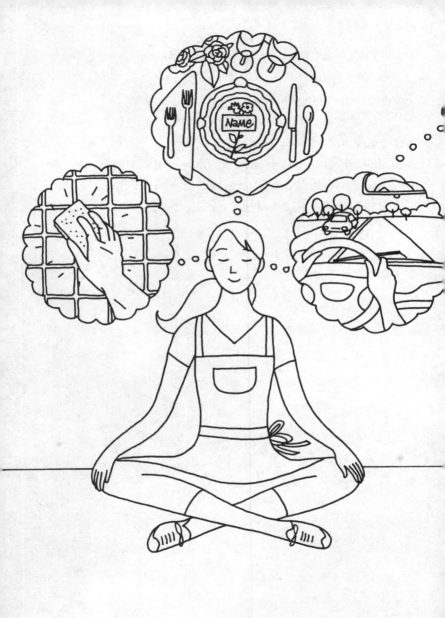

Section Three

BEING PRESENT

Chapter 17

Entertainment

For as long as history has been recorded, theater and entertainment have been a cornerstone of societies and cultures. Of course, the platform has changed a bit—only a few years ago, formalized entertainment was generally held in organized theaters and meeting points. Now, it seems that even the youngest of children have their own personal entertainment devices that allow access to entertainment at their fingertips. While many people worry (with good reason) that this constant access to media is detrimental to healthful meditation, there are ways to engage in entertainment—movies, music, television, and social media—without allowing it to take over your life

Have you ever seen a great movie that was so captivating that you lost yourself for the duration of the film? I went with my wife to see the final part of the Hunger Games series, *The Hunger Games: Mockingjay - Part 2*. Since we don't like crowds, we opted to go to the movies on a Sunday at 9:30 A.M. and found a scarcely filled theater. The movie was excellent. At no point were either my wife or I thinking about what we needed to do later that day, what time it was, or anything else. In fact, my wife came to tears many times during the movie. It was so captivating, it freed our minds from all other thoughts, responsibilities, and worries.

We spend so much time living our own lives that it is sometimes wonderful to live through the eyes of another. This is exactly what movies are able to do for us. For adrenaline junkies, high-stimulation, action-packed films can offer an escape without the risk of actual dangerous situations. For those who would like to lighten up their mood and get the endorphins going with some laughter, we have comedies. And for those folks who may need to feel better about their own lives, a drama could help them realize their own lives aren't so bad and things could be worse.

Live-theater performances can also provide a temporary escape. By ducking into a theater to see *Finding Neverland* or *Les Misérables*, Kathy and I left our own lives behind and lived vicariously through the characters onstage. As a result, we were able to face whatever we had in front of us feeling more refreshed, rejuvenated, and overall just a little bit happier.

The same goes for professional sports, although the dynamic is different. Since the original Olympics of ancient Greece and the gladiator games in ancient Rome, people have come together to enjoy and spend time watching competition. I once took my mother to a New York Yankee playoff game. It was my mother's favorite pastime, and growing up in New York, we always had

Yankee games on in the house. The experience of watching the game with thousands of die-hard fans who were focusing their full attention on what was happening on the field allowed me to forget what was going on in my own. I was able to experience the energy and passion of Yankee Stadium. When the Yankees won, people were crying with joy.

You may have seen avid sports fans yelling at the top of their lungs at their big-screen TVs when their team either won or lost. Maybe you yourself do this. If you do, you probably feel as if the team is an extension of yourself—and by connecting yourself with something outside of you and your own mind, you can achieve a meditative focus.

As long as your mind, body, and spirit are focused on a single activity, you will achieve active meditation. When you wholly embrace a movie or performance, you are able to turn off your mind and temporarily escape from the craziness of life. It is an opportunity to recharge your batteries, just like with more traditional forms of meditation.

We only have a certain amount of mental energy to spare. Once the energy is depleted, our ability to handle stress and challenges decreases. This is when small situations can become crises—when stress is present and the slightest mishap will throw you off. This happens when we don't function on all cylinders, and we make poor choices as a result. The only way to replenish diminished energy is to recharge your batteries, just as if you were to plug in your cell phone at night. Seeing a show or going to a ball game that takes your mind off things for a while is an opportunity to do so.

One thing to be sure of is that you choose a movie or form of entertainment that will allow you to escape. A while back, my wife and I were with my good friend Master Melella and his wife Gina at our home in Vermont. We decided to see a movie. There were two choices: a comedy, or Chris Kyle's story, *American Sniper*. Everyone opted to see *American Sniper* except for me—I opted to see the comedy. It's not that I wasn't interested in *American Sniper*—I was—but I chose the comedy because I didn't want to watch a movie that I had to think about. I just wanted to enjoy a show. We did see *American Sniper* that evening, and it was an incredible movie; it was remarkably thought-provoking and a truly powerful story. It was exactly the type of movie that I did *not* want to see at that time. I was looking for a light-hearted, fun movie. There are times for serious and powerful movies, and although I would have definitely seen *American Sniper* at some point, I would have preferred to see it when I was mentally able to process it.

In one sense, *American Sniper* kept me consumed because I wasn't thinking about anything else at the time, so I did experience some meditation. The movie continued to consume my thoughts after it was over, when all I wanted to do was enjoy myself. When I watched *The Hunger Games: Mockingjay - Part*

2, it was a different story. My conscious mind turned off during the show and reactivated once the movie was over. It's important to find a movie that will disengage your mind and allow it to rest and recharge.

Many people debate whether visual entertainment is a form of meditation, or simply another activity that requires focus. Some believe that if you engage in outside stimulation to calm the mind, it cannot be considered meditation, mainly because meditation should come from within. I believe watching a movie or engaging in visual entertainment are both forms of active meditation; however, it must begin with the right intention. If you intend to watch a movie and distance yourself from reality, then you will experience meditative benefits, providing it is engaging. If you choose to watch a thought-provoking movie, then it most likely will not be a meditative experience, because it will keep you focused throughout. Enjoy a movie for the sake of enjoyment without the need to invest too much of yourself in the movie, and you will gain some meditative benefit.

It is important to note that an occasional movie, play, or even sports event is an extremely healthful form of mental escape, but not too often, as it could become counterproductive to your mental and spiritual development.

Chapter 17 Key Points:

- Don't allow constant online access—television, movies, social media, etc.—to take over your life.

- When you engage in any form of entertainment, be sure to mentally prepare and separate all other facets of life from the experience. Be present and mindful and take it all in.

- Involve friends and family. It is always great to see a movie, play, sports event, or any other form of entertainment with someone else who will enjoy it, too.

- While dramas definitely have their role, nothing is more beneficial than an uplifting and inspiring form of entertainment. Be sure to engage in entertainment that is going to reflect the experience you wish to have.

Chapter 18

Cooking and Cleaning

When I went to Korea for the first time in 2000, I had an opportunity to spend three days at a Buddhist temple and sleep among the monks. We slept on hardwood floors with a four-foot by four-foot block of wood as a pillow. Accommodations were Spartan, but the beauty and tranquility of the temple far outweighed the uncomfortable arrangements.

Every day at the temple, resident monks did their chores. No matter the task, they executed it efficiently and effectively. They looked at their everyday chores as part of their training. They wouldn't simply do the chores to get them done as fast as they could in order to go on to the next thing; they did them with a high sense of pride as they mindfully engaged in the task. They took pride in everything they did, and it showed—from the gardening of the grounds to the care of the temple, and especially in their food. Whether they were preparing food or doing household chores, their minds, bodies, and spirits were engaged in the activity, which enabled them to be in a constant state of meditation. Mindfulness threads through everything they do as they live their lives for spiritual development.

Take a moment to reconsider the idea of active meditation as we've been defining it. Instead of working toward "mindfulness," imagine aspiring to "mindlessness." We all do many day-to-day tasks that don't require much thought but still have a meditative benefit. These mindless activities are quotidian responsibilities, like household chores, laundry, food shopping, cooking, and all of those necessary but not always pleasurable tasks. My wife often comments how certain activities are very calming for her, so she doesn't mind them at all. For example, she loves to cook. I, on the other hand, don't necessarily look forward to laundry, but find myself fully engaged in the task of doing it when it's required. I do it out of necessity and survival to an extent, and the action of putting clothes into a washer and dryer isn't especially enlightening to me—but folding requires a physical mastery that tends to lead to a pleasurable freedom of thought that often has me stopping to write down unexpected new ideas.

Cleaning, too, can be a mindless activity with surprising benefits beyond a spotless house. It is easy to clean the house or a room and then find your mind wandering to a place completely unrelated to the task. You may also notice that the satisfaction and calm that comes with living in a clean environment can be conducive to a clear mind, which, in turn, is more receptive to meditative states. You will find yourself sleeping better and waking up more alert and open.

My brother-in-law (who I call Uncle Gus) is a retired Marine who spent a great deal of his career working on and maintaining all sorts of helicopters for the military. This can be a stressful job, because if you make a mistake, lives could be on the line. Uncle Gus is a very skilled guy. He is extremely mechanically inclined and does beautiful carpentry; he created such a beautiful home that I believe he could have a great second career working on houses. But instead, after he retired from the Marines, he began working at a local grocery store, stocking shelves very early in the morning. When I asked him why he chose to do this instead of using his skills to get a more advanced job, his response was "Because it's mindless work, and I needed to clear my head."

Gus said that because he spent so much of his career as an active Marine working on helicopters and making sure they were safe and ready to go, he needed to decompress. Stocking shelves was an opportunity to make a few extra dollars and have a job that didn't require him to think. It didn't come with the responsibilities and the pressure of his past career, and that allowed Gus to take the time he needed to plan the next stages of his life. He is now contracted by the military to manage the mechanics that have the same responsibility that he had when he was a Marine, so ultimately he did go back to his old routine of constantly thinking on his feet and being responsible for the lives of others. However, the thinking he did while engaging in the relatively mindless task of stocking grocery shelves gave him the opportunity to reconsider his life without external distractions or pressures.

Mindless work doesn't need to be limited to household chores but could be anything mundane that offers the opportunity for meditation.

Chapter 18 Key Points

- Being mindful of the task at hand will allow you to fully appreciate what you are doing and find peace in every activity.

- Stress and pressure can cause you to rush through the tasks haphazardly. Allow yourself the time to engage fully in the experience. It makes a world of difference.

- Remember, the atmosphere surrounding the task also creates a meditative experience, not just the task itself. Play music or calming sounds.

Chapter 19

Driving

People have been driving cars since the release of the Ford Model T, the first production vehicle released in 1908, created and envisioned by the famous Henry Ford. Henry Ford had the vision to create an "automatic mobile" which we now call the automobile. He is also the author of one of my favourite quotes: "Whether you think you can or think you can't, you're right." Henry believed that he could put mainstream America in automobiles just as Bill Gates believed he could put personal computers in everyone's home. The automobile has evolved so much since the early twentieth century.

In a 2016 study, the Federal Highway Administration reported that males drive an average of just over 16,500 miles per year and females drive an average of just over 10,500 miles—that is a lot of time spent in cars. With all that time to burn through, driving can certainly become a meditative experience.

Have you ever been driving and found that ideas just began coming to you? Have you ever experienced a situation while driving where the solutions to challenges you were facing presented themselves? Have you ever been on a long drive and found yourself listening to an audiobook, podcast, or the radio, and it put your mind in a different place even though you were still driving? If you answered "yes" to any of these questions, then you have been in an active state of meditation while driving.

Driving is one of those mindless activities that allow the mind to wander and drift while still performing effectively. People utilize the time in their car in various ways. Some people listen to music—my personal favorite pastime while I drive is to listen to spa or meditation music.

Others listen to podcasts, which have brought a whole new element to driving. I personally have come up with a lot of business ideas by listening to podcasts. There is literally a podcast for any interest—not just for business development, but also for specific hobbies, interests, personal development, and anything else you could possibly imagine.

Audiobooks have a similar benefit and offer the opportunity to lose oneself while driving. I remember when the final Harry Potter book came out, my wife and I purchased the audiobook and listened to it with our family as we drove to and from Vermont to go snowboarding. It made driving that much easier, and, better yet, it allowed my children to use their imaginations instead of playing video games or watching movies.

If you have a lot on your plate, driving can be a time to allow yourself to sort through any issues, identify priorities, and make plans for tackling problems. Ideas may spontaneously come to mind, and you may find that using a recorder or your smartphone to capture the idea is a good way to remember everything you think of. I, like many, have used Apple's Siri feature to assist in making notes. In the past—when Siri was unavailable—I pulled over and made notes in a notebook to capture a thought.

When you are driving, you are of course engaged in the task in the same way as when you are walking, but a veteran driver doesn't *have* to purposefully ponder through every decision unless there is a hazard that requires him or her to change strides—the skill is embedded in the subconscious mind. That is why I refer to driving as a "mindless" activity.

There is, however, a difference between driving "mindlessly" and letting your thoughts wander while still paying attention to the road. As I've mentioned previously, being distracted and passively consuming information is different from maintaining attention while also entering into a meditative state. It is impossible to enter into a meditative state while on your phone and driving (which you should never do, as it is very dangerous). It could be argued that it is impossible to enter into a meditative state while playing on your phone—period.

My home in Stowe, Vermont, offers the best snowboarding,

skiing, hiking, and mountain biking on the East Coast (in my opinion). However, it is a five-hour ride from my home in New York. I have a ritual that helps make the drive go by very fast and makes the trip enjoyable. Once I cross the Vermont border, which marks two hours remaining on the trip, I put on the soundtrack for *Les Misérables*. The music is so soothing and the story is so powerful that I thoroughly enjoy the music and the ride. My mind escapes, it seems like effortless driving, and next thing you know, I have arrived at the house. My daughter is currently a student at the University of Vermont in Burlington, just forty-five minutes north of Stowe, and when she travels back home on occasion, she does the same thing. In fact, now when she drives her friends, they end up singing *Les Misérables* together on the drive. It helps make the long ride pass quickly and makes for an enjoyable experience.

Please look at driving as a time to give yourself an opportunity to lose yourself in whatever you choose. Driving is a mindless activity that is embedded in our subconscious because we have done it so often in our lives. Every time you drive your car, you are able to benefit from the ride as a form of active meditation.

Chapter 19 Key Points:

- While driving, always stay aware of your surroundings to ensure safety for yourself and other drivers.

- Promote a calming atmosphere. To allow your mind to be calm, put on spa- or meditative-style music to create an environment that relaxes you.

- Meditative experiences while driving may bring on valuable thoughts and ideas. Carry a recorder with you or use your smartphone to capture meaningful thoughts.

Chapter 20

Prayer and Faith

Many years ago, when I was on a journey to advance my spiritual training, I came to a very meaningful realization. My mother was dying—her airway had become blocked and she was in the ICU with no hopes of making a recovery. My brother, sisters, and I were comforting each other and trying to make sense of the situation in our own way. I remember sharing a section of the book *Living With the Himalayan Masters* by Swami Rama with them. In section *XIII: Mastery over Life and Death*, the chapter "Birth and Death Are but Two Commas" talks about how the spirit (1) is present before we arrive physically at birth and (2) lives on after death. It was comforting for me to hear and gave me the feeling that my mother's spirit would live on. Because I was both the youngest of four and the only sibling involved in martial arts and spiritual training, my brother and sisters half accepted and half dismissed this concept. However, at my mother's memorial service, our childhood pastor offered this message: "Don't look at Ann's passing as the end; look at it as a comma in her existence. . . . Her spirit will live on forever." My brother and two sisters looked at me in amazement because it was exactly what I had shared with them.

This was also around the time when I finished training with an energy master to help increase my own internal ki energy and open up necessary channels to do so, including my third eye (for a refresher on ki energy, refer back to Chapter 11: Moving Meditations on page 110). The third eye is a heightened intuition that enables one to see things beyond what physical sight allows.

With the events of the service and the quest for my own personal spiritual development, I was inspired to pick up a copy of the Bible and start reading it. To my amazement, its words resonated with me in a way they never had before. As a young child, I had been very involved in my local church. My sister and I would walk to Grace Lutheran Church every Sunday and were actively involved in the youth program. When my family moved away, we stopped attending. Shortly after, I started my tae kwon do training and established a new network of friends in the martial arts community. Being a history major in college, I was always intrigued about how religion shaped the world's history, but it was purely an interest on an academic level, not a spiritual one. It wasn't until my mother passed away that I was able to find the true essence of religion and how it related to my own spiritual development.

Mathew 6:22 in the King James Bible reads, "The light of the body is the eye: if therefore your eye be single, your whole body shall be full of light."

It was this verse that merged many elements of life into one for me. It made clear that my spiritual development and my religious development were one and the same. Before I read this verse, I never saw these two paths emerging as one.

To put it simply, I have been training for years and hours on end to open my third eye and have heightened intuition in order to serve my students and clients better. When I read that verse, I realized that what I have been pursuing is the same spiritual path that people search for through religion. It brought together on one path two worlds that I thought were so far apart. I learned and realized that the spirit that runs to and through us in meditation is the same as the Holy Spirit. My training has included prayer ever since I read the verse.

But prayer in meditation isn't relegated to the Christian or Catholic variety—you may find that you have similar revelations when you immerse yourself in spiritual material from a variety of disciplines. You don't need to have been born into a particular faith to experience the benefits its teachings can impart. Exposing yourself to a wide variety of religions will provide you many avenues to explore in seeking the kind of clarity I've been describing as a meditative experience.

One of my closest friends and my third partner in Empowered Mastery is Nick Palumbo. Nick owns and operates a successful financial-services company and is also a principal in our coaching company. Nick has done very well for himself over the years; I believe he is the true definition of success. He has a wonderful relationship with his wife, great relationships with his children, he finds time to exercise regularly, and he is successful in his career.

Nick shared his daily routines with me and explained how he has developed a relationship with God like no other. When I spoke to him about meditation, he shared that he practices prayer meditation in every waking moment, seven days a week, 365 days a year. Prayer meditation requires tapping into your personal relationship with the higher power of your choosing. It has nothing to do with any specific religion or faith; it has to do with your own personal relationship. Swami Rama said it best in *Living with the Himalayan Masters*:

> All the great religions of the world have come out of one truth. If we follow religion without practicing the truth, it is like the blind leading the blind. Those who belong to God love all. Love is the religion of the universe. A compassionate one transcends the boundaries of religion and realizes the undivided, absolute reality.

The reality is this: The sole relationship you have with your creator is much more significant than the faith that you follow or believe in. Prayer meditation continuously strengthens that relationship, no matter your religion.

To Nick, the difference between religion and prayer is that religion educates and prayer connects. Meditative prayer is the personal relationship you have with your creator, your spirit, the supernatural, or what many people refer to as God. It takes you beyond the physical—or even intellectual—plane and gives you the ability to tap into a spiritual place that many don't even know exists.

The desire to practice meditative prayer came from Nick's search to find something larger than himself. At Empowered Mastery, we always talk about our "life's purpose" and ask our clients what the purpose of their lives might be. In Nick's world, there are two purposes: a primary and a secondary.

Nick's primary purpose in life is to know God and love God. His secondary purpose is his own individual intentions and the personal road map he sees for his life. "The only way to know and love God is to talk to Him. He gives you the answers because He designed you—no one else did. He designed you with a purpose, for a purpose that allows you to fulfill the purpose He set for you," he explained.

During our interview, Nick revealed that he has been practicing prayer meditation for four years at a meaningful level. Before that, he practiced what he called "selfish prayer," where he prayed solely for his own personal gain. As he described, those prayers were a "me, me, me moment" of what God could do for him. He added, "Now it is about how God could use me for his purpose."

Nick consciously practices meditative prayer all the time, from the moment he wakes up to when he goes to bed. When we discussed this, he referred to a quote from Denzel Washington: "I pray that you all put your shoes way under the bed at night so that you gotta' get on your knees in the morning to find them, and while you're down there, thank God for grace and mercy and understanding."

Nick is always asking himself, "What's the lesson I need to learn?" He likened the experience of speaking to a higher power to that of having your best friend with you all the time. "When I pray, it is as if I am sitting next to [God], having a conversation in a car."

Dr. Wayne W. Dyer, an internationally renowned author and speaker, once said, "If prayer is you talking to God, intuition is God talking to you."

Nick went on, "God shows you the way, and when you have a personal relationship, everything starts to become clear. You start to accept things that you think are challenges and obstacles because you know that it is by His design and He is molding you to be who He wants you to be. When you understand this, you tap into the same energy source we always talk about at Empowered Mastery. You have tapped into your creator and you become one with God. You begin to do things that you once thought impossible—He is never going to let you down."

Nick once had a huge house and nice cars, and took exotic

vacations, but he always felt something was missing. When he learned what prayer and a relationship with God really meant, he knew he would give it all up if needed.

Nick shared with me two instances where he realized that the relationship he has with God was more substantial that he could have ever imagined:

> I was in Napa Valley with my wife and a bunch of colleagues and good friends. We went to a beautiful winery overlooking the valley. It was a time in my life when I had a lot of doubt. My father was sick, and I was preparing for his demise. There was a lot of pressure on me. I couldn't figure out the lesson that I needed to learn. I was by myself having a great glass of wine, and I remember looking at the mountains and saying, "God, I remember there was a time in my life where I was on top of the mountains. But now I feel like I am in the valley. What's the answer, God, why do I have to feel like I am in the valley for this long?"

> I got home on a Sunday, and I got a phone call at 7:30 A.M. from my good friend Gino. Gino says to me, "How are you, my brother?" First thing comes to my mind is, What does he need from me? Does he need money, a favor, what does he need? Gino replied these exact words: "God put you in my heart today and told me to tell you something—I don't know why I felt the

urge to call you this morning—but God told me to tell you that it is always greener in the valley." Gino never knew what thoughts were going through my mind when I was in Napa.

The second story happened at a Ranger game. It was around the same time, and doubt kept settling in. I was constantly having these moments where I was asking God, Why do you keep challenging me this way? I said to my friend, "I am wondering at this point whether God even exists," and my friend called me out and called me a hypocrite. He said, "You always told me to trust in God and now you're not trusting him, so you're a hypocrite."

I thought to myself: What do you know? You are not going through what I'm going through. I got to my car at ten o'clock that night after the game, and I received a phone call from my good friend Gino again. "My brother, I need to talk to you," he said. "You know I never ask you for anything, right? But I need a favor. Promise me that you'll do this for me."

I thought that perhaps he needed money. I said to Gino: "Anything. Whatever you need—I'll help any way I can."

Gino replied, "God told me to tell you to trust in Him."

Nick pulled over on his way home and sat there on the shoulder of the road, crying. He called Gino the next day and explained what had transpired, and Gino's reply was, "I know, I can't tell you how I knew, but I knew I needed to call you. I can't tell you why, I just knew."

Gino has a special relationship with God and has transformed countless lives through his mentorship and advocacy. No matter where Gino goes, he shares his faith and inspires others to follow his example. He is a good person who will go above and beyond to help anyone in need—a true believer of the power of love and compassion. Once, when I was talking to Gino, he was talking so passionately and with so much certainty, he gave me goose bumps all over my body. Gino said, "Those aren't goose bumps, those are God bumps—you have been touched by God."

Prayer meditation involves taking the time to allow God to come into your life. Nick said it is about "surrendering" to Him, so of course I asked Nick to elaborate.

"Surrender is giving up control. It's about asking, 'What is the lesson that I need to learn today?' Everything that happens— good or bad—is by design. Why? Because He is building you up for something bigger. It's human nature. The more successful you are, the more in control you think you are. You think you're in control, but He is sailing that ship, not you. Surrender is putting yourself in a sailboat in the ocean with a huge storm and saying to God, 'Please get me through this,' and trusting in Him to get you through the storm. That is surrendering to God," explained Nick.

He continued: "It is about having unyielding faith. We all know that faith is the belief in the unknown. Real faith is the relationship. It's knowing that He is present in me. Even speaking right now, He is speaking through me to you in this conversation.

"Even when I read the Bible, I ask God to give me the ability to read and absorb it at a spiritual level and not only in the flesh. In the past, I would read in the flesh. Now when I read it, I find the solutions to every challenge I may have in life. It's all in there. Prayer meditation is tapping into a higher energy, which is my creator. It's realizing that everything in existence has started way before my time."

Nick's favorite verse is from the Bible, Romans 12:2: "Do not conform to the ways of this world, but be transformed by the renewing of your mind. Then and only then will you know me."

Nick's suggestion for anyone who is looking to use prayer meditation as a means to establish a relationship with God is this: "One needs to be wholeheartedly present when in prayer for it to have full meaning and intention."

It's as John F. Kennedy said in his 1961 Inaugural Address's most famous lines: ". . . ask not what your country can do for you—ask what you can do for your country." It's not what God can do for you, but what you can do for God.

In order to develop a strong relationship with a higher power, you will have to pray with your mind, body, and spirit. It may not involve kneeling or even putting your hands together—a prayer can be wherever and whenever you wish, as long as you are submitting yourself fully to what you are doing and feeling with 100 percent conviction and unyielding faith.

This is prevalent in all major religions. In Judaism there is a great deal of Torah and scripture readings. Prayer meditation is achieved when you are embracing the meaning and essence of the scriptures and not just reading them at a superficial level, but rather taking in every word and finding the deeper understanding of the message and how it relates to the relationship you have with God. Jewish spiritual leader and Torah life coach Frumma Rosenberg-Gottlieb's March 13, 2011 "On Mindfulness and Jewish Meditation" article explained, "Prayer is an advanced form of meditation; yet it is also simple and accessible to all. The Hebrew word for prayer, *tefilah*, implies connecting to and bonding with one's spiritual source. In fact the prayer book, the *siddur*, can be seen as a highly sophisticated, structured guide to cultivating our awareness of the presence and the power of G-d."

Islam has the same purpose of meditation as all other religions—to strengthen the relationship between man and God. Emil Ihsan-Alexander Torabi, creator of the Islamic Meditation Program—an online training program to enhance Islamic spirituality—wrote the following on his blog, *Islamic Renaissance*:

Meditation in Islam is turning inward, and thus away from the world created by the human ego, seeking to discover rather the Divine Presence of God, subtle and superior to the illusion of *dunya* [*dunya* translates to "world"].

The Islamic Prophet Muhammad wrote in his scriptures, "One hour of meditation is more valuable than seventy years of obligatory worship." You see, prayer meditation is all about the relationship with your creator. It doesn't matter what you call your creator or whether you are Islamic, Jewish, Catholic, Hindu, Sikh, Wiccan, Mormon, Christian, or any other type of faith. What matters is that you are genuinely 100 percent committed to your own personal relationship with God.

I asked Nick to share a meditation prayer that he uses in his own life. Feel free to adjust it to fit your own beliefs and preferences.

Father God, thank you for your mercy and your grace. Thank you for your love, thank you for not only what you have done for me in my life but what you are about to do in my life. I pray for my family, I pray for my wife and my relationship with my wife, my relationship with my kids, and my whole family. I pray for those who need prayer in their lives. I pray for my enemies. I want more of you and less of me all the time. I want to surrender my heart to you, and please, forgive me for my sins. Show mercy for me and my family.

Chapter 20 Key Points:

- It doesn't matter what you believe. What matters is your personal relationship with your creator.

- When praying, be sure to commit your entire mind and spirit to the prayer. Distractions will take away from the meaning and intent of your words.

- You can pray in any place or at any time, but one of the most powerful places to pray is in an environment that you have created specifically for prayer. Creating a personal prayer sanctuary in your home or going to an organized religious space can serve as an opportunity for meditative prayer.

CONCLUSION
Always Be Meditating

Thank you for giving me the opportunity to guide you on this journey. I hope you've gathered some information about how to incorporate active meditation into your life. For some of you, this may be a whole new outlook on meditation.

As you may have picked up throughout reading this book, the type of meditation I have been referring to is a mindset rather than an action. The action of meditation is the act of doing without thought. My true hope and wish for everyone who reads this book is that you approach everything you do by being fully present and mindful at all times.

You may remember the 2002 *Spider-Man* movie starring Tobey Maguire and Kirsten Dunst. Do you remember when the school bully attacks Peter, and Peter's "spidey senses" make the punches seem as if in slow motion? Peter is easily able to dodge, and even admire, them, as if from a third-person perspective.

When you are mindful, you will view life in this way. Actions and events appear as if narrated from a third party. You may feel like an observer looking in on your own life. This state of being could happen *to* you and *for* you all the time, anytime. All you have to do is be mindful of each moment and keep your thoughts aligned with what you are doing.

So, in short, how can someone practice meditation all the time? It is both easy and challenging at the same time. Easy—all you have to do is be present. Challenging—it is very difficult to be present all of the time. The objective is to be consciously aware of the current moment and what you are doing; at that point you will always be in a state of meditation.

I was a young parent, only twenty-three years old when my oldest son was born. As he got older, I would take care of him in the morning, take him with me to tae kwon do, and my wife would pick him up after she got home from work. I remember lying on the rug with my son and his Thomas the Tank Engine train set; we were completely present and wholeheartedly engulfed in the moment. Nothing else mattered to either of us for that moment in time. It was pure bliss. I was mindful of my son in that moment, and nothing else in the world mattered. That is just one instance of a meditative moment that came about because I was spending time mindfully.

My challenge for you is to find as many opportunities to experience true mindfulness as you can. Free yourself from distractions by living your life as if you are always in a state of meditation. No matter what you are doing, you have the ability to be in a constant state of meditation. I can tell you firsthand that you will be calmer, possess more inner peace, have more meaningful relationships, take your profession to a whole new level, and not let other people, circumstances, or events affect how you feel. You will be a much happier person overall.

Thank you for the opportunity to serve you!

With love and respect,
Chris Berlow

INDEX